Suzanne Lavoie
NATUROPATH

SO YOU THINK YOU'RE *Healthy?*

LISTENING TO YOUR BODY
AND DISCOVERING THE
12 PRINCIPLES
FOR GETTING AND KEEPING
GREAT HEALTH!

SO YOU THINK YOU'RE *Healthy?*

Copyright © 2017
Suzanne Lavoie

Printed in Canada

All rights reserved. No part of this publication may be reproduced, distributed or transmitted in any form or by any means, including photocopying, recording or other electronic or mechanical methods, without the prior written permission of the author, except in the case of brief quotations embodied in critical reviews and certain other non-commercial uses permitted by copyright law. For permission requests, email author at: **soyouthinkyourehealthy@gmail.com**

DISCLAIMER

The content of this book is for general information only. You should never delay seeking medical advice, disregard medical advice or discontinue medical treatment because of information in this book. If you have any specific questions about any medical matter, you should consult your doctor or other professional healthcare providers.

Library and Archives Canada Cataloguing in Publication

Lavoie, Suzanne, 1959-, author

So You Think You're Healthy? : Listening to Your Body and Discovering The 12 Principles for Getting and Keeping Great Health / Suzanne Lavoie.

Includes bibliographical references and index.

Issued in print and electronic formats.

ISBN 978-0-9947475-0-1 (paperback)

ISBN 978-0-9947475-1-8 (pdf)

ISBN 978-0-9947475-2-5 (html)

1. Self-care, Health--Popular works. 2. Medicine, Preventive-Popular works. I. Title.RA776.95.L39 2015   613   C2015-904217-8
                                                                                  C2015-904218-6

To contact the author, visit
www.suzannelavoie.com
www.soyouthinkyourehealthy.com

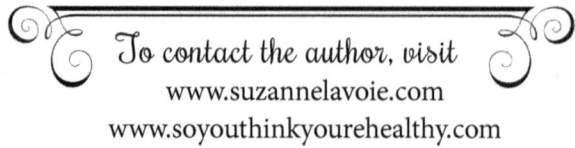

S.L. Publishing

Praise for SO YOU THINK YOU'RE *Healthy?*

"Very good book! It will help thousands of people… if not more. We are a nation of sick people. In fact we human beings are the sickest living creatures on this planet. The question is why? Perfect health cannot be purchased in a bottle of pills. Perfect health is the result of a healthy lifestyle. People needing to know more about how to achieve health and vitality, no matter what their age, is central to the health message of this book. Here we have a person who believes in the health message, and this book is her gift of love to the world. Now, dear reader it's up to you to experience a life of endless energy and perfect health."

~ Christian Limoges, Naturopath, Clinique L'Aube

"Suzanne states the unhealthy lifestyle issues clearly and guides us with proven, whole-person principles and action steps that we can easily apply to greatly enhance the quality of our lives. A must read for all who seek wellness."

~ Denis Waitley, Author of *The Psychology of Winning*

"This is a timely explanation with disease at an all-time high. Suzanne Lavoie has successfully written a user-friendly guide to educate all of us on how to lead a healthier lifestyle."

~ Leigh Erin Connealy, M.D., Author of *The Cancer Revolution*

"This book offers a wealth of knowledge for people searching for explanations to the many possible causes and solutions to modern day illnesses. Bravo to Suzanne Lavoie for courageously tackling this massive and vitally important subject."

~ Miranda Esmonde-White, *New York Times* best selling author of *Aging Backwards*
Creator and Co-founder of Essentrics® and Classical Stretch™

"Health is an absolute priority for everyone and Suzanne's wonderful book will help you recognize how you can experience optimum health, greater energy and clearer thinking. This book dives deep into the understanding that every reader needs to know to… quite simply, have good health. If good health is something you desire, make this book your one resource."
~ Peggy McColl, The Millionaire Author Maker

"There are many who believe that we must be content not to be sick in order to be... healthy. In this book, Suzanne guides us to a more exciting vision for optimal health, one that takes into account all of the human parameters through a healthy and conscious lifestyle. Thank you for helping us to love who we are and to believe that we can aim higher and farther."
~ Murielle Matteau and Daniel Ladouceur,
Founders and Directors of Centre Option-Voix

Dedication

In loving memory of my beloved brother Roch.

*To my family and friends and all who have lost loved ones
to a degenerative disease.*

*To my children: Jérémi and his wife Carine, Josef, Kristof and Caleb,
and to your future wives-to-be and all your future children.
May you live a prosperous, healthy life.*

Let food be thy medicine
and medicine be thy food.

– HIPPOCRATES

Contents

- 9   FOREWORD
- 11   PREFACE
- 15   INTRODUCTION

---

17   *Part One*: GETTING TO THE ROOT OF OUR ILLNESSES

- 19   *Chapter 1*
  THE BASICS OF NUTRITION

- 39   *Chapter 2*
  EXCITOTOXINS, PHTALATES AND OTHER TOXINS

- 67   *Chapter 3*
  HOW THE BODY CLEANS ITSELF

- 87   *Chapter 4*
  DASHBOARD LIGHTS AND DEGENERATIVE DISEASES

- 111   *Chapter 5*
  A RADICAL CHANGE TOWARDS GOOD HEALTH

131 *Part Two*: A HEALTHIER YOU

133 *Chapter* 6
THE 12 PRINCIPLES TO GUIDE YOU BACK TO GREAT HEALTH

157 *Chapter* 7
GETTING STARTED

175 ABOUT THE AUTHOR
177 ACKNOWLEDGEMENTS
179 RESOURCES
181 ENDNOTES
191 OFFERS

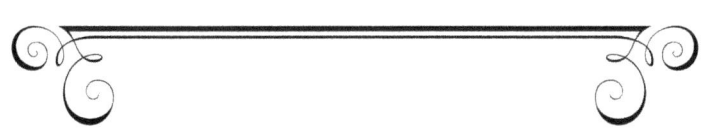

Foreword

This book, *So You Think You're Healthy?* is a must-read for anyone who has even the slightest interest in health. Most people have sorely neglected the stewardship of their physical bodies, and are not aware that they are abusing and starving their bodies of required nutrients. Many seem to believe that chronic, degenerative diseases mysteriously come out of nowhere and randomly afflict and kill people. This shows a lack of understanding of sowing and reaping patterns. God designed our body to function in health and to heal itself from external attack when given the proper care and nutrition it was intended to have. If you have been one who has wondered why so many today are afflicted with sickness, please read this book and discover clear answers.

Most people think, "If I don't have cancer, high blood pressure, or diabetes, and I eat a pretty 'healthy diet,' I'm okay." In this book, you will find many things you did not know that are essential for true health and avoidance of chronic degenerative disease. You'll encounter a lot of "Aha" moments. Suzanne has done a masterful job of explaining in very simple terms how our body functions and the basic principles of becoming and remaining healthy. You will discover 5 major factors contributing to the formation of degenerative diseases, ignored by most people.

It is impossible to fulfill your destiny from a grave or a life of pain, sickness and chronic, degenerative disease. If you believe in your destiny and that of your family around you, please don't forfeit the completion of your God-given assignment on earth due to a lack of knowledge of the proper stewardship of your physical health. I highly recommend this book as a foundation for understanding the basic principles for maintaining good health.

Craig Hill
Founder of Family Foundations International
www.familyfoundations.com

Preface

During the period of my life when I was struggling with my health, I did not know why I was sick. The doctors didn't know what was wrong with me, either. My body, however, was telling me loud and clear that something was wrong. I was overtaken with fatigue and exhaustion a good part of the time. Normal life just had to be put on hold for a while. I was perpetually questioning myself: What is wrong with me? Why I am so tired? What is going wrong inside my body?

I slowly began to get some answers and to understand how everything is connected. I began to realize how the type of food I ate really did make a difference. I could also see how my thoughts and emotions played a role in my quality of life, and how buried emotions from hurts in the past could actually affect my health today. I went on to experiment in several ways to get healthy results in my body. My curiosity led me to read more and more books, and I began to attend conferences and to take courses on health and healing.

During this period, my friend became sick with cancer. She had her ups and downs: she went into remission after having spent some time at a world-class health center, but soon relapsed and started going downhill. I so wanted to help her! I felt deep down that there was something I could do. I was unable to communicate what I felt so deeply about: that a radical food change and an emotional examination were important to her healing. Unfortunately, a short time later she passed away.

As time went on, I saw several acquaintances pass away and more and more people around me succumb to different diseases. I remember especially one professional person with a powerful life message who was speaking at a conference. He spoke with passion and intensity, and taught the audience about how we needed to live our lives in a proactive way. In the midst of his powerful and fervent teaching, he fell on stage and, in front of 10,000 people, died of a massive heart attack. Seeing people die from diseases in the prime of life was disturbing. By now I could no longer contain the conviction that was steadily rising up in me: *What they are eating is not providing them with proper nourishment, I thought, but they aren't aware of it; and who I am to say anything?* Because of this strong belief that kept growing in me and because of my wonderment of the human body, I eventually undertook professional studies to become a naturopath. A naturopath is a professional who deals with sickness and disease through foods, plants and herbs. I also continued learning about the healing of our emotions and how that can have a tremendous positive effect on our physical body.

The more I gained knowledge and understanding of what goes on in the human body and in our emotions, and even the connection between the two, the more I wanted to help others with their health problems. However, I wasn't sure how to go about doing so. It was only after my mentor and coach, my beloved brother, died of cancer that I got up the courage to act and do what I could to help anyone willing to listen and learn. That is when I decided that I would write this book explaining why we get sick and what we can do to regain our health, inspired by what I have picked up through my studies, observations and through my own life experiences.

Having gone through my own different life challenges, I have come to appreciate the wisdom acquired in enduring difficult times. The beauty of facing obstacles in life is that if we have learned and grown from these painful events, errors and even miserable situations, we can then teach, train and pass on our knowledge, life experiences and new-found knowledge to others; in doing so, we help make this world a better place. We can have the satisfaction of knowing that, perhaps, we didn't go through these things for nothing.

I have also come to the conclusion that if we don't take preventive measures to keep our body healthy, in our later life, if we become weak and frail, we won't have that passion and energy to pass on our experience, knowledge and wisdom to the next generation. Our children are then left going through trials and errors that could have been avoided if we mentors had been there to guide them and train them. Mistreating our body, even though we may be unaware of doing so, and succumbing to disease or premature death as a result, is unfair to us as well as to our children and grandchildren. This is an urgent call to wake up.

In addition to raising awareness of the multiple consequences of neglecting our health, I try to use simple explanations and create images that you can use to support your understanding in order to help you make changes that will, in turn, bring you healthy results. Actually, whether you understand or not, I guarantee that your body will react instantly to the healthy changes that you start to make and will begin to work immediately to bring about restoration and health. When you are convinced of what you need to do and act upon this, you will put yourself in an environment where your food and lifestyle choices are more positive.

In short, Part 1 of this book has been written to help you demystify the illnesses of our modern society and Part 2 to establish steps and principles that you can follow in order to put everything on your side to be able to live a healthy, energized, productive life.

Introduction

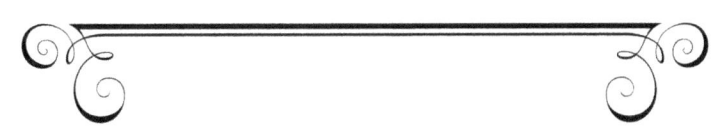

I had my first warning signs of illness many years ago when I was still single. I distinctly remember one particular year when I had several bouts of terrible sore throats. I would be bedridden for several days and hence missed quite a few days of work. I had taken five or six prescriptions of antibiotics throughout the year. Towards the end of this time, I really started questioning myself as to why I was always so sick. One of the roommates I was living with at the time often made caramel fudge. I was addicted to sugar and was always the first to dive in to have my fill. I started experimenting with my consumption of this sugary treat and finally made the connection. I realized that I would always get sick right after binging on this delicious candy.

I got married a short time later. I asked my husband to please help me with my sugar addiction because I never wanted to get sick the way I had the previous year. We made an agreement that neither of us would buy any processed sugary foods, like cakes and cookies, but would allow only homemade whole wheat raisin bran muffins. I was chronically constipated and thought the bran would help. Secretly, I thought it would be a good way to still indulge in my sugar addiction, only in a healthier way.

I was not aware of what a really healthy diet was. Naturally, I cooked and ate the way I had learned to while I was growing up at home. It was a pretty good diet in the sense that we weren't exposed to a lot of junk food or soft drinks, and having been raised on a farm we were able to benefit from a lot of fresh, organic garden vegetables, and for this I am very grateful. The problem for me was that I ate way too many carbohydrates like bread, cakes and cookies. I developed a tenacious carbohydrate addiction.

Following the birth of my first child, I was a wreck. My doctor had no idea what I had. Even though no official tests were done, I diagnosed chronic fatigue and the beginnings of fibromyalgia* as my problems. I had aches and pains everywhere all the time. It got so bad that I would have to take at least two days to recuperate after making the humongous effort of taking my baby to his medical checkups. If I vacuumed my house one day, I was knocked out the next with pain and crippling fatigue, unable to do or undertake anything. It was a very challenging and discouraging time of my life.

One day, I overheard someone talking about a *bio-nutritionist*. I had never heard of this type of profession before and was intrigued. I got her phone number and called her up. My slow journey to taking back my health had officially begun. In addition to my personal appointments with her, I began to assist some of the classes she gave periodically. I started learning about things I had never heard about before. I initially had no idea what caused me to be sick. With her teaching I began to realize that I indeed was unknowingly doing some things that contributed to my pain and illness. I began understanding the basic principles of how food works in our body and what causes our body to get run down and prone to disease. With her guidance, I threw out all of my processed food and began my journey of learning about eating real food. This was a turning point in my life. This began my quest for understanding what role nutrition plays in preventing disease.

We tend to disassociate from what we don't see or understand. I believe it is very important to get informed as to what goes on in our body. With a bit of knowledge and understanding, we become empowered. And, if we choose, we can do our part to make our body function optimally and thus actively taking charge of our health. Through this book, I hope to inspire you to start making those healthy changes now, and a little bit every day.

Let's begin our journey together.

---

*musculoskeletal pain

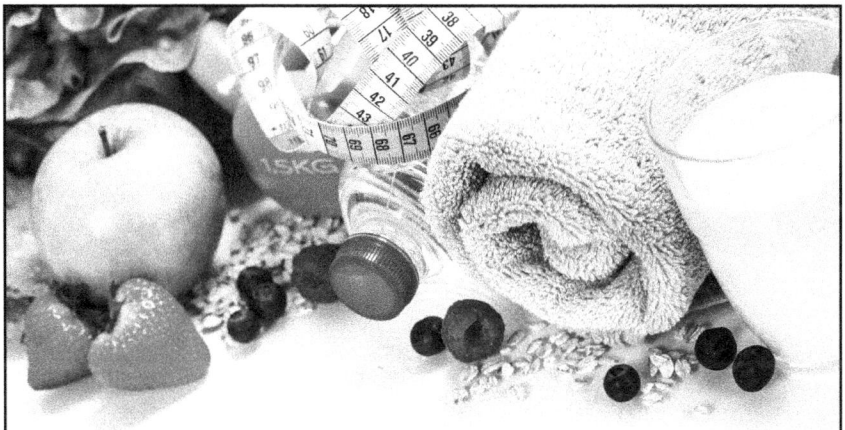

PART ONE

Getting to the root of our illness

We get sick because we are not aware of the terrible ways that we treat our body. We come down with various illnesses because, without realizing it, we fuel ourselves with food that lacks the necessary nutrients to rebuild bodily structures. Additionally, we consume and inhale toxins daily. This degrades the body, making us even more susceptible to illness and degenerative disease. In this first part of this book, I provide an overview of our nutrient-deficient diets and the consequences this has on our health. I also expose the many toxins prevalent in our environment and how our body deals with these toxins, and how stress, living a sedentary lifestyle and negative emotions can contribute to our dis-ease.

1
CHAPTER ONE

The basics of nutrition

Let's compare our body's metabolism and its digestion process to the burning of wood in a woodstove. The metabolism in this analogy is the stove, the wood is our food, the heat from the fire is the energy in our body, and the ashes and smoke symbolises fecal matter and other toxins. When we eat food, or put a log on the fire and it is digested or burnt, this creates energy and leaves behind "ashes" and residue that then must be evacuated. When we eat processed foods (packaged foods, fast foods, canned foods and even certain cooked foods), the digestion process not only leaves behind ashes (fecal matter) but also toxic residue. Consuming these foods leaves our body with the huge chore of cleaning out these toxins. What's more, when we regularly eat these low-quality foods, we deprive ourselves of necessary nutrients to effectively nourish and heal our body.

The serious nutrient-deficiency problem facing this present generation is also caused by the way food in the majority of "developed countries" is farmed, processed and marketed on a mass scale. Because the food industry is so compactly controlled, it may seem as if we – the consumers – have little to no choice. But with knowledge and proper guidance, we can choose the right kinds of food and learn to avoid foods that harm, rather than heal, our bodies. Together, as we make more and more of these healthy consumer choices, the food industry will necessarily have to adjust to this growing demand.

HOW WE NOURISH OURSELVES THROUGH DIGESTION

If you want to be proactive in gaining better health, first you must observe and understand how you are nourished. So let's take a closer look to see what is happening inside our bodies.

For the most part, we are nourished by the digestion and absorption of the food that we eat. First the food gets crushed up in our mouth with our teeth. The enzymes in our saliva further break down the food. Once it reaches the stomach, the chewed food is turned into a sort of mush through the gentle kneading of our stomach muscles along with the aid of different gastric juices. Hydrochloric acid, a strong gastric acid, helps break down meats and other proteins. It also protects the body from illness by killing pathogens that are often found on the foods we eat.

The food, which has now been transformed into a sort of purée called *chyme*, is now ready to leave the stomach. This chyme receives more digestive aid as it enters the first part of the small intestine where it will be treated with more enzymes and insulin produced from the pancreas. At the same time, bile from the liver via the gall bladder, acting like a soap, emulsifies the fats.

The transformation of the food, after having passed the first part of the small intestine has more or less completed the digestion process and has liberated the molecules of nutrition to be absorbed and then assimilated by the body. Our body needs to absorb and assimilate many different kinds of molecules for it to remain healthy: calcium, magnesium, carbon, hydrogen, potassium, sulphur and sodium – to name a few. Many other trace elements are also required, for example zinc, copper and selenium. These minerals, vitamins and trace elements, also called micronutrients, are required for optimum health.

Most of these nutrients are absorbed through our small intestine. The small intestine has many tiny folds that increase the surface of absorption. These tiny folds are covered with *villi*, tiny finger-like tubes that are covered with very minute hair-like tubes called *microvilli*. These microvilli capture food molecules from the chyme found in the small intestine. These molecules of nutrients get transferred into the villi tubes which also contain tiny blood vessels called *capillaries*. These nutrients, once absorbed through the capillaries are then carried away through the blood stream to be made available to every one of our cells, nourishing all the different parts of our body.

What is important to remember is that nourishment actually happens on a cellular level. That means that whenever you are eating, it is your cells that you are feeding, not your stomach.

Once the nutrients have been absorbed from the small intestine, this chyme then proceeds to the large intestine where we find beneficial bacteria that will break down and ferment fibre. A particular type of fibre called *prebiotic*, once fermented, becomes an important food source that will nourish and help proliferate beneficial bacteria. This healthy gut bacteria, also known as *probiotics*, in addition to having a great impact on overall immunity, aids in maximizing the absorption of certain nutrients in the colon.

Another function of the colon is to extract the water from the chyme leaving behind fecal matter that will then be excreted from the body. The water removed from the large intestine is reabsorbed and recycled by the body, thus contributing to its level of hydration. There you have it: the basic steps of digestion.

> NOURISHMENT HAPPENS ON A CELLULAR LEVEL

This, hopefully, helps give you a way to peek inside your body to get an idea of what happens to the food you put into your mouth. Again, what is important to remember is that it is your cells that are being nourished. Your body is made up of trillions of cells. These cells are the basic building blocks of everything else in your body. They make up your organs. If your cells are not well nourished, then your organs cannot be healthy. And if your organs are not healthy, you are not healthy either. As complex as the body is, the fundamental principles from which we can live by to ensure healthiness are really very simple.

OUR BODY IS DEFICIENT IN NUTRIENTS

One reason we get sick is because of nutritional deficiency. If our body is missing some necessary element, over time it can be compromised, and we then become susceptible to disease.

In the Western world we might think that nutritional deficiency is caused by not getting enough to eat. After all, we have all heard of people dying of starvation in underdeveloped countries. We have a lot of food available to us, so it's inconceivable for most of us that we could be undernourished. However, if we don't eat the proper foods that contain the many and varied elements that our body needs to function properly, then, yes indeed, we can become malnourished. If we eat food that has poor nutrient content, even if the body does digest it, the elements the body needs to rebuild and nourish itself properly are not all there. Over time, regularly eating low-quality foods with low vitamin and mineral content can cause nutritional deficiency.

To better understand nutritional deficiency in the human body, let's use as an example the construction of a house. To build a house, you need various kinds of building material. You need wood to build the frame of the house, drywall panels to erect the walls, electrical wires covered with protective sheath to carry electricity, pipes for the plumbing to evacuate the sewage, glass windows to let the sunshine in, shingles on the roof to keep the water out and bricks to keep the inside of the house comfortable and safe-guarded from the external elements.

What would happen if you didn't have enough wood for all of your framing needs? Or if the wooden frames were of inferior quality, twisted and split? Or if you used thinner framing wood instead? How about if you didn't have enough drywall? And what if the wiring had sections without protective covering? Your house would not be very sturdy nor would it be very secure. It would not withstand the test of time.

> OVER TIME, EATING LOW-QUALITY FOODS WITH LOW VITAMIN AND MINERAL CONTENT CAUSES NUTRITIONAL DEFICIENCY

Your Body Is Your House

You need to take care of your house by offering it all kinds of good-quality building material. If you want a good, sturdy foundation of health, you must be proactive when it comes to choosing the food that goes into your body. Yes, it takes a certain level of commitment to do this, but the benefits are so worth it. If you are young, you might not see any physical evidence of a poor diet. However, with time you will reap what you have sown – or in some cases what you haven't sown. Take care of your future health by nourishing yourself with proper nutrients today.

The nutrients that are required by our body are divided into two major categories: *macronutrients* and *micronutrients*.

MACRONUTRIENTS

Carbohydrates, proteins and fats are all considered macronutrients. These macronutrients provide the calories in our diet which in turn give us energy. They are also required for growth and other metabolic functions our body needs to function on a daily basis. They are present in larger quantities than micronutrients.

CARBOHYDRATES

Carbohydrates come from plant foods. Whole, non-refined carbohydrates are healthy carbs. We can divide carbohydrates into three different categories: *sugary or sweet carbohydrates* like fruits; *starchy carbohydrates* which include all grains, certain root vegetables and legumes; and *non-starchy or fibrous carbohydrates* which encompasses all other vegetables, including green, leafy vegetables. Please note that things like pastries, cakes, fruit juices and soft drinks are all *refined sugary carbohydrates*. Pasta, bread and crackers are *refined starchy carbohydrates*. Our body transforms all carbohydrates into glucose molecules that produce energy. Carbohydrates are the easiest macronutrient to be transformed into energy.

PROTEINS

Meats, fish, poultry, dairy products, eggs, nuts, seeds and legumes are all sources of protein. The body uses proteins, which have been digested and broken down into amino acids, for the construction of its structural parts, such as muscles, organs, nails and hair, as well as aiding in tissue repair. Proteins also aid in immune function and help create hormones. Hormones are messengers that send signals to tell the body to initiate different actions, such as producing digestive enzymes, initiating fat storage, breaking down and releasing fat or initiating the menstrual cycle in women.

FATS

Cold pressed olive oil, raw nuts, avocados and wild Alaskan salmon are excellent sources of healthy fats. Saturated fats are also excellent fats but for many years have been wrongly criminated against. Coconut oil, palm kernel and palm oil (certified sustainable) are other sources of beneficial fats. Fats from meat, butter and cream are also healthy sources of saturated fats, particularly if they come from grass-fed animals. Baking with, or frying foods in non-hydrogenated, minimally processed lard, as opposed to refined vegetable oils, is far less detrimental to our health. These types of saturated fats, although often blamed for causing diseases, are healthy and necessary; our body cannot thrive without them. Sugar, refined carbs, refined vegetable oils* and trans fats, as we will cover in the following section, are what cause weight-gain and heart disease, not saturated fats.

The fats or lipids we consume, particularly saturated fats, are used in the construction of cell membranes, the protective part of the cell, and so remain a very important macronutrient. Fats are responsible for the transporting of fat soluble vitamins A, D, E and K. They are crucial in promoting a healthy metabolism, provide energy, and aid in immune health. Additionally, healthy fats, which include saturated fats, support heart and brain function, our brain being made up of a good percentage of fat and cholesterol. Saturated fats are needed for mineral absorption and many other biological processes. Fats are also used as an insulator and help protect our vital organs.

*pro-inflammatory omega 6 oil

A WORD ON TRANS FATS

Trans fats are vegetable oils that have been transformed by industry. Because freshly extracted oils from vegetables turn rancid very quickly, food scientists have discovered that adding extra hydrogen molecules to vegetable oil increases the stability of the oil thereby prolonging the shelf life of the food containing these oils.

Consuming foods that contain trans fats wreaks havoc in our body, and they can actually block the healthy benefits of good fats. Staff from the Mayo Clinic have stated that doctors consider trans fat the worst kind of fat you can eat.[1] The body does not recognize the molecular structure of this type of fat. They cause oxidative damage to our cell membranes, which causes inflammation, leading to all kinds of degenerative diseases. We must avoid all consumption of trans fats.

A big problem is that these trans fats are in a lot of the foods we regularly eat. They are in most pastries, crackers, frozen pizza crusts, almost any packaged flour product including cakes and cookies, peanut butter and in many deep frying oils and therefore in most commercially fried foods. They can be found under the name "hydrogenated oil" or "partially hydrogenated oil" in the ingredient list and "Trans Fats" or "Trans" in the Nutrition Facts Table. Be careful however, as certain governmental laws allow a small amount of trans fat to be in a product but not on the label because of a certain method of rounding off a number to zero for a food product containing less than 0.5 g. per portion.[2,3] Beware, these "portions" do add up!

> THE FOODS WE LOVE TO EAT ARE OFTEN LOADED WITH TRANS FATS – MAKING IT IMPOSSIBLE TO KEEP OUR BODIES HEALTHY

IN SUMMARY

Unfortunately, most of us have not been trained to differentiate between healthy and unhealthy macronutrients. We often eat refined carbohydrates that lack fibre and important trace elements. In addition, we eat too much poor quality meat: hormone boosted and treated with antibiotics, or processed meats containing nitrates and other preservatives. We are also consuming an overabundance of bad fat. Consequently, we are not receiving the good nutrition our body needs. We are being invaded with toxins coming from the consumption of these low quality foods, making it impossible for our body to remain healthy. Furthermore, the overconsumption of refined carbohydrates, as well as too much animal protein – both void of fibre – leads to constipation and to general congestion in our body.

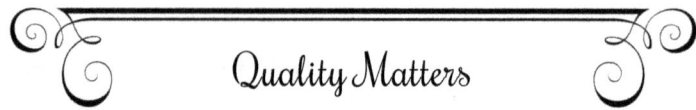

It may seem apparent that as long as we are eating carbohydrates, proteins and fats, even if they are of low-quality, our body will keep us alive and active since macronutrients provide energy. However, this is somewhat of an illusion because if the fats, proteins and carbohydrates are not of good quality – that is to say they are void of micronutrients (see next section) – eating them will actually contribute to the weakening of your body, thereby setting you up for disease. Yes, you may be alive and moving, but wasting away from malnourishment on the inside.

MICRONUTRIENTS

To fully understand nutritional deficiency, we need to look at the second category of nutrients called micronutrients. These are minerals, vitamins and the very important, but often unrecognized, antioxidants and phytochemicals. These nutrients are present in the body in much smaller amounts and in general don't provide energy but assist in many important functions in the body.

Phytochemicals* for example, are chemical compounds that occur naturally in plants. Thousands of different phytochemicals have been discovered in food, particularly in fresh fruits and vegetables. They have many desirable properties for sustaining health in our body, including antioxidant activity.

Antioxidants are desperately needed to combat the production of ever-increasing free radicals** that damage the cells in our body at a molecular

---

* "phyto" meaning plant
** molecules with unpaired electrons which rob other molecules of their electrons

level. Stress, pollution, toxins, chemicals and the digestion of poor-quality foods produce free radicals. Damage from free radicals on our delicate cell membranes as well as on the structural components within the cell are known to be at the root of degenerative diseases and premature aging.[4]

We cannot underestimate the importance of these micronutrients. When we eat a sandwich, which is composed of macronutrients, we can't see the micronutrients (vitamins and minerals) it may or may not contain. Obviously, we see the bread. We know it is food, so we eat our sandwich not asking ourselves if it contains the micronutrients that our body requires.

Many times we eat foods that taste good to our palate and fill our stomachs, but much of this food contains what is known as "empty calories." These macronutrients provide calories, which produces energy and gives us a feeling of satiety, but they don't necessarily give us good nutrition. On the other hand, consuming many micronutrients keeps at bay nutritional deficiency. The types of foods that contain abundant micronutrients are whole foods; that means non-processed foods, particularly raw fruits and vegetables, sprouted seeds and nuts.

NUTRIENT LOSS IN OUR SOILS AND PRODUCE

Plants can generate vitamins and enzymes, provided that they are exposed to the proper growing conditions, as well as to the proper nutrients in the soil, but they can't produce minerals. Minerals must be absorbed from the soil. If the soils are depleted, the plants therefore don't contain the minerals that are needed for the proper construction of our body. Our soils today are greatly depleted.

A study by Dr. Donald R. Davis conducted by the University of Texas, collected data regarding declining fruit and vegetable nutrient composition. He states the following: "Recent studies of historical nutrient content data for fruits and vegetables spanning 50 to 70 years show apparent median declines of 5% to 40% or more in minerals, vitamins, and protein in groups of foods, especially in vegetables."

The magazine *Scientific American* published an article citing various other studies depicting soil depletion. For example, a British study looked at nutrient loss in 20 vegetables between the years 1930 to 1980, while the

Kushi Institute did a similar study with 12 vegetables between the years of 1975 and 1997.[6]

1930 TO 1980		1975 TO 1997	
BRITISH FOOD JOURNAL		**KUSHI INSTITUTE**	
Average nutrient loss of 20 vegetables		Average nutrient loss of 12 vegetables	
Calcium	19% loss	Calcium	27% loss
Iron	22% loss	Iron	37% loss
Potassium	14% loss	Vitamin A	21% loss
		Vitamin C	30% loss

The declining of nutrients in our soil began in the 1940s and continues to do so up to our present day. So why is this happening? Today's major agro-farm companies do not farm the land the same way farmers have in the past. Years ago farmers periodically used a summer fallow method to let the soil replenish its minerals. They also used crop rotation so that the same minerals would not be removed from the soils year after year. As crops grow, they absorb nutrients from the soil. When crops are harvested, so too are the nutrients absorbed by the plants. This leads to a cumulative loss over the years.

THE THREE KEY MINERALS

In today's high-yield farming, to continue to grow abundant crops year after year, commercial farmers use fertilizers to return to the soil three key minerals: nitrogen, phosphorus and potassium. Nitrogen is a key element in protein. Often used in greater amounts than other nutrients, nitrogen helps make plants green and plays a major role in boosting yields. Phosphorus provides the energy for plants to thrive and the energy that a plant needs to grow, while potassium helps plants fight stress and disease, and to grow strong stalks.

The utilization of only these three minerals produces big healthy-looking plants, but they don't provide the many other minerals we need to stay healthy. We also need calcium, sodium, magnesium, sulphur, boron, copper, iron, manganese, molybdenum, nickel, zinc, silicon, cobalt and selenium – and more.

Modern farming techniques create healthy-looking plants which lack the nutrients we need to maintain healthy bodies

According to some scientists and doctors, our body needs more than 80 different nutrients in order to achieve optimal health.[7] It is obvious that these would be difficult to attain from our depleted soils. And when you consider that many fruits and vegetables in our grocery stores have come in from long distances, sometimes from half way around the globe, it's impossible not to have some depletion of vitamin content along the way. However, this in no way means that eating fruits and vegetables is not important. It just means that we ought to put in a more conscious effort to ensure we ingest more vitamins, minerals and other important nutrients.

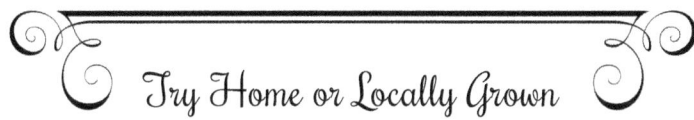

Try Home or Locally Grown

One way of ensuring that you are eating nutritious, pesticide-free food is by growing your own food or by starting a community garden. Everyone should try to grow some kind of garden, even if you start by growing parsley in a pot on the kitchen windowsill. It is also a good idea to consume as much locally grown produce as possible. The nutritional content of these foods is much higher. Not only that, but by buying locally, we encourage our precious local farmers.

Currently there is a rising awareness on the benefits of eating organically grown foods, free of pesticides. These types of crops are known to have a higher vitamin and mineral content and are normally free from genetically modified organisms (GMOs). Eating organic is of course optimal, but unfortunately not in everyone's reach yet. Hopefully, in the future it will be increasingly possible to find organic produce at a reasonable price. Keep your eyes open for discounts. Opting for organically grown foods whenever we can will eventually make them available at more affordable prices. Don't hesitate to make a request for organic produce from your grocer. Eventually, more and more of our local farmers will be able to meet this growing demand. If eating organic is not accessible to you at this time, please don't think it to be absolutely necessary. The benefits of eating non-organic fruits and vegetables far outweigh not eating them at all. Using vegetable washes can at least help to remove the chemicals on their skins.

Scientists may be able to quantify how many minerals and vitamins vegetables and plants contain. However, they are not able to completely identify or explain all of the functions that the trace elements, phytonutrients and antioxidants play in our body. So even if our vegetables and fruits are depleted of many minerals and vitamins, we need to eat them every day because there are many other benefits that we are unaware of that contribute to healthy bodies.

Consuming fresh, raw foods also provides us with certain digestive enzymes. Enzymes are vital for sustaining life and serve a wide range of important functions in the body. They act as catalyzers and significantly speed up the rate of virtually all of the chemical reactions that take place within cells. They are known to catalyze thousands of biochemical reactions, including the digestion and metabolizing of foods. Enzymes provided from our foods prevents us from depleting the ones our body produces. From these facts alone, it is evident that we need to consume much more of these raw foods than we have been accustomed to.

Furthermore, solely taking into consideration the beneficial factors of the fibre from raw fruits and vegetables keeps us heading in the right direction. Fibre helps in reducing cholesterol build-up, controlling weight gain, lowering blood glucose levels, detoxifying our body and ensuring proper bowel transit. Eating raw and cooked vegetables and fruit daily is very important.

In addition, because of today's age of fast-paced living, high stress levels, increasing free radical damage, as well as being over-exposed to so many all too convenient fast foods, it is of utmost importance to complete our diet with a daily intake of a good quality supplement. This provides your body with a broad spectrum of vitamins and minerals as well as antioxidant capacity. Adequate intake of micronutrients are fundamental to having a healthy body.

THE BASICS OF NUTRITION | 31

You can trace every sickness, every disease and every ailment to a mineral deficiency.

~ Dr. Linus Pauling
Two-time Nobel Prize winner

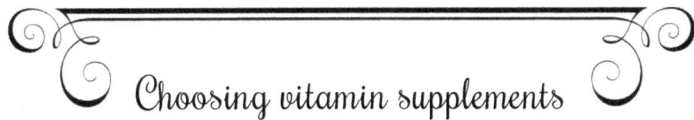

Choosing vitamin supplements

When choosing a vitamin supplement, exercise caution. Some vitamin supplements are actually harmful for you. An article in GreenMedInfo stated that leading brands of children's vitamins contain aspartame, a sugar substitute which has at least 40 adverse side effects, including brain tumours. These vitamins also contain other harmful substances such as cupric acid, zinc oxide, hydrogenated oils, sorbitol and genetically modified corn starch.[8]

Be vigilant and do your homework before choosing any kind of supplement. Rely only on top-quality products that have been researched and verified, rather than those that are unproven or unreliable. Beware of being influenced by advertising hype and deceitful marketing strategies. Consult the *Comparative Guide to Nutritional Supplements** found in bookstores to help guide you in your choice of top-quality supplements.

GENETICALLY MODIFIED ORGANISMS

Genetically modified foods are banned in a lot of European countries; in North America, however, they do not even need to be labeled. We may be inadvertently consuming more than we think. The Institute for Responsible Technology provides us with a few reasons to avoid genetically modified organisms (GMOs)

> **GMOs are unhealthy.** *According to the American Academy of Environmental Medicine (AAEM), GMOs can contribute to organ damage, gastrointestinal and immune disorders, infertility and rapid aging in animals.*

---

* McWilliam, Lyle. (2017) *Comparative Guide to Nutritional Supplements*. USA: Northern Dimensions Publishing. 6th Edition

GMOs may cause long-term health problems. *For instance, the genetic modifiers used on GM soybeans have been known to transfer into the DNA of the bacteria living inside our body. Insecticides in genetically modified corn have been identified in the blood and foetuses of pregnant women. For these reasons, the AAEM encourages doctors to prescribe non-GMO diets for their patients.*

Genetic engineering creates dangerous side effects. *Combining genes from entirely unrelated species can result in a number of unpredictable side effects. This is partly because the process introduces foreign information that can produce toxins, allergens, carcinogens and nutritional deficiencies within the body.*[9]

Let's make a concerted effort to request the labelling of all genetically modified foods so that we can be better informed, permitting us to choose the quality of the food we consume.

DAIRY

Dr. Campbell, in his book *The China Study* makes reference to Dr. Hegsted, a scientist with remarkable experience in calcium research. This scientist stated in one of his papers "…hip fractures are more frequent in populations where dairy products are commonly consumed and calcium intake is relatively high." He also points out, regarding a study involving 10 countries, that a higher consumption of calcium was linked to a higher risk of bone fracture. He specifies that in this study, much of the calcium intake indicated on the chart was due to dairy products rather than calcium supplements or non-dairy food sources of calcium.[10] As we can see, we don't necessarily get an adequate intake of calcium through milk products. There are several reasons for this:

- The intense pasteurization that commercial milk goes through makes it insoluble, therefore rendering unavailable most of the calcium found in raw milk. It also kills the good bacteria.
- Milk is a protein and proteins are acidic. Eating lots of dairy puts the body in an acidic state. The body neutralizes this acidity by leaching out its own calcium from the bones, carrying it to the blood in order to maintain the required acid-base balance. When our body remains in a prolonged acidic state this also causes inflammation which we will talk about in more detail in chapter 4.

- Older people develop difficulty digesting milk because their enzyme bank that digests milk gets more and more depleted as they age.

Other points on the draw backs of drinking milk:

- The molecules in cow's milk are bigger than our human bodies can properly digest. We are often left with small particles of undigested milk lingering in our body. These extra undigested proteins can cause milk allergies or milk sensitivities.
- Many people have an intolerance or sensitivity to milk products and are not even aware of it. This may be causing them symptoms such as: skin rashes, sinus problems, bloating and even diarrhoea.
- Industrial dairy cows are constantly being injected with hormones and antibiotics to keep their production of milk high and to help curb epidemical outbreaks. Not to forget they are also being fed GMO corn and soy, which has all of its own detrimental side effects. Therefore, when we consume these dairy products, we are also exposed to these same harmful substances.
- Milk also produces large amounts of mucus in our body. I drank milk myself when I was younger, and I always had an annoying accumulation of mucus in my throat. I constantly needed to clear my throat. When I went off milk products, the mucus in my throat also disappeared. If you come down with a cold, dairy is one of the first things to be removed from your diet.

It's interesting to note that we are the only mammals that drink milk after weaning. In other words, only babies need milk to survive.

I strongly believe that as adults we are better off not drinking industrialized cow's milk at all. If you live in this society, it's hard not to be continually exposed to industrialized dairy products. If you want to eliminate or cut down on dairy, but you're having a hard time, choose only raw cheeses and natural yoghurt with no added ingredients. Raw and fermented milk products do have certain benefits. Kefir, for example, is a beneficial probiotic and it can easily be made at home. You can exchange cow's milk with other healthy alternatives, such as almond milk, rice milk, coconut milk, non-GMO soya milk, cashew milk or even raw goat's milk. Goat milk's protein molecules are smaller and thereby easier to digest than cow's milk.

In all honesty, I never gave cow's milk to my children while they were growing up. They didn't get much ice-cream or cheese either. I certainly don't regret it. Most ice-creams are loaded with toxic additives, never mind the quantity of added sugar. I have four boys, all very adventurous, and they have had their share of accidents. Some of them have been hospitalized several times after attempting acrobatic stunts and ensuing tumbles, but thankfully, not one of them has had any broken bones.

You may still argue that we do get calcium from milk and that milk is good for you, but our family is living proof that you don't need milk or its products to receive the calcium you need. We just haven't been taught that calcium is also found in certain fruits, in plants such as nettles, in vegetables – especially in dark green, leafy vegetables – and in most seeds, particularly sesame seeds.

FEEDING OUR CHILDREN

The most critical time to ensure healthy eating is without a doubt in early childhood. Being proactive during this time has a twofold effect. First, it lays the foundation for healthy eating habits that normally follow a child for the rest of its life. Educating our taste buds by savouring tasty, natural foods is a powerful antidote to consuming processed foods. Moreover, taking the time to eat in a relaxed and pleasant environment is a key factor for good digestion and thus ensures a better absorption of food nutrients.

Second, because this is the period when the body develops and grows the most, the body of a child is therefore in need of good quality material for construction. Vitamins, minerals and other essential nutrients are crucial for the duplicating cells that are in the process of creating healthy structures such as bones, muscles and organs. Healthy cells ensure a good foundation for the future, and they provide children with resistance to illness later in life. Undeniably, good, healthy food lays a solid foundation for future health.

It's horrifying to observe what certain small children and even some small babies eat: French fries, chips, candy, commercial desserts, sugar-loaded juices and deep-fried chicken or fish sticks. Remember, these foods often contain dangerous trans fats. Additionally, food industries market products like Froot Loops® and Nutella® as containing healthy vitamins and minerals to make us think that these foods are healthy. Young children eat so many of these processed foods that they have absolutely no taste or desire for eating any real food like vegetables. Even the peanut butter we buy for our kids is detrimental because it contains trans fats and added sugars. When shopping for any kind of nut butters, look at the labels, and make sure they have no trans fats or partially hydrogenated oils – or sugar – added to them.

How can our children possibly stand a chance of having a healthy adult life when they are ingesting processed, nutrient-devoid, toxic-laden foods at such an early age? The danger with our kids eating all of these processed foods is that the fibre of their growing bodies will be made up of these low-grade materials. Remember the example of the construction of our house? If we don't have good building materials to start off with, the house will not be as resilient and will fall apart sooner. As adults, we along with our parents and grandparents, have had – for the most part – a healthy start. Chances are that 40, or even 20 years ago, while some of us were still growing, we had access to much healthier whole food; much more nourishing than what many children eat today. So we have a head start or a cellular advantage, so to speak, because the genesis of our cells was healthier, and duplicated using good construction material.

> GOOD, HEALTHY FOOD IS A MUST FOR LAYING A SOLID FOUNDATION FOR FUTURE HEALTH

AGING TOO SOON

Many of today's children carry a toxic load right from the start of their lives. Can you imagine what the future holds for some of these kids who in addition to this have been eating junk food all their lives? Their organs are made of tissue whose foundation lacks the vital nutrients necessary to reproduce healthy cells that resist disease. Their cells are already in an age-stricken state despite their young age. Additionally, they suffer premature accumulation of toxins and incur damage typically found in most people of advanced age.

The article "Young Kids, Old Bodies" cited the case of a child called Kimberley Rhodes. Because of scars created by layers of fat, Kimberley's liver no longer produces healthy levels of necessary enzymes. At only 13 years of age, this young child's health mirrors that of nearly two-thirds of adult Americans who are overweight or obese.[11] She is already considered pre-diabetic and at risk for hypertension. She is not alone. An ever-increasing number of children are consuming tonnes of empty calories.

THE DANGERS OF EMPTY CALORIES

Empty calories contribute not only to lack of nutrients but also to childhood obesity, which leads to diabetes and other serious diseases. Some of today's younger generation, who are stricken with these diseases, are even dying sooner than their parents.

Passing on healthy habits includes more than just monitoring what our kids eat. They also need to consume lots of good quality water. Kids, as well as adults, tend to drink lots of fruit juices or soda pops that contain no real health advantage. These juices are usually filled with sugars or artificial sweeteners that are sometimes worse than sugar. Even so-called healthy juices can raise blood sugar levels, which causes high blood sugar issues. In addition, when kids drink these juices in abundance, they act as fillers, thereby cutting down their appetites for healthy food. We can train ourselves and our children to regularly enjoy drinking pure, clean water.

A TEACHABLE MOMENT

Whenever my kids get sick – yes, they do occasionally get sick – I always find it is the best teachable moment to instill principles and truths about how their bodies work. I use these moments to teach them how to interpret signs and symptoms and to look for root causes to their problems.

Our youngest still goes to school and takes his lunch with him every day. I have to credit my husband for making most of his lunches, and I assure you that for the most part they are healthy and creative! In the late fall, he somehow stopped filling up our son's metal thermos bottle with pure, clean water. I'm not sure exactly why, but I started asking him if he was drinking enough water. His response was always, "Yes, Mom." I kept reminding him, "Remember, as soon as you get home, drink a big glass of water before you eat anything else. Let that become your lifelong habit."

One day he came to me and said that he had pain on the top of his head and he didn't know why. It was a sharp, aggravating pain. I had just found out that it had been several weeks that he was no longer bringing his water bottle to school, and I knew he was getting dehydrated. I told him so and encouraged him to start drinking more water again. Well, of course, he didn't – he had gotten out of the habit.

Several days later, on his last day of school just before his long anticipated holidays, he came down with an intense fever and became very sick. He was unfortunately too sick to attend his Scout party that evening. What a disappointment! Did he drink water that night and the next day? You bet! He was on the right track, including drinking warm herbal teas. Did he feel like eating junk food? Nope! He wanted a warm vegetable soup made from homemade chicken broth. He said, "Mom, it's amazing that our body often tells us what we need to eat." I told him, "That's right, our body does tell us what we need to eat, but sometimes we don't listen and let our taste buds overpower the message."

> OUR BODY TELLS US WHAT WE NEED TO EAT

I asked him if he had learned something from this experience. Yes, he will drink more water and bring his water bottle to school every day. It's quite reassuring to see that he is now measuring his water intake daily.

SUMMARY

- **Start paying attention.** Many of the whole foods that we do eat have far fewer nutrients today because of the way that high-yield farming depletes the soil. This has resulted in nutritional deficiencies without our realizing it. Without bringing awareness to the food that we eat and taking a critical look at how it has been produced or cultivated, we are making ourselves – and our children – vulnerable to vitamin and mineral deficiency. Choose organic, non-GMO foods whenever possible. It is also important to consider supplementing your diet.

- **It's time to wake up.** We have allowed ourselves to blindly consume low-grade processed food products, such as processed meats, refined carbohydrates and all kinds of fast foods, too many industrial dairy products, sugars, commercialized juices, trans fats, and without our knowing, some genetically modified foods, thereby setting ourselves up for future disease instead of intentionally providing our body with nourishing macronutrients and micronutrients.

- **Make better choices.** Looking at how we nourish ourselves and choosing healthy whole foods, with the awareness that we are in fact feeding our cells, our tissues and our organs, are crucial first steps on the pathway to health.

Let's take a look at how the many toxins we are exposed to affect our body.

CHAPTER TWO

Excitotoxins, phthalates and other toxins

Many of the toxins that enter into our body are there without our knowledge or conscious consent. These include agricultural pesticides, harmful preservatives, other chemicals found in our processed foods, toxins found in personal care products and perfumes, sprays and cleaning products, prescription drugs and toxic levels of heavy metals found in fillings and vaccines. There are also toxins that are generated by our negative emotions and stress. With increasing awareness of our surrounding environments we become empowered to make new healthy choices. Avoiding, or at least greatly decreasing exposure to unsafe chemicals, helps reduce damage incurred on our physical and mental well-being. In the same way, as we become more conscious of our negative inner thought processes, we can choose to gradually replace harmful thoughts with positive ones. We can also begin implementing proactive measures to combat chronic detrimental stress.

AGRICULTURE

Agriculture today is not what it used to be. In the past, farms were smaller. Farmers didn't use chemical fertilisers or pesticides, but rather relied on traditional ecological ways to ensure healthy diversified crops that would resist devastation provoked by impoverished soils and insect infestation.

Today's mass farming methods are detrimental to the earth. Industrial farming's goal is the mass production of food in the shortest amount of time for increased profits. It does not use proven natural techniques, such as crop diversification, which prevents the soil from being demineralised. Rather, the same crops are planted year after year. This monoculture farming impoverishes the soil and makes it susceptible to erosion, as well as weed and insect infestation.

This kind of mass farming relies heavily on artificial fertilizers and chemical pesticides. These agro farmers may also fertilize their soils with manure. However, this manure is often contaminated with bacteria. This is because the cows are fed and fattened with corn. According to the documentary *Food, Inc.*, consuming a diet rich in corn products creates acid-resistant *E. coli* that lives in cow manure.[1]

These bacteria, artificial fertilizers and chemical pesticides can get into the run-off as well as the underground water systems. Nearby communities which tap into the surrounding bodies of water are being adversely affected in their health, contributing to serious diseases. According to the Pesticide Action Network (PAN), the pesticides, insecticides and fungicides used on our food are proven *endocrine* (hormone) disrupters, affecting men, women and children alike. These chemicals have an adverse effect on the reproductive system causing birth defects, miscarriages and stillbirths.[2]

A news broadcast in Seattle reported that a local lead researcher at Fred Hutchinson Cancer Research Center, Dr. Kristen Upson, and her team, observed 248 women who had recently received a diagnosis of endometriosis, declaring the following:

The take-home message from our study is that persistent environmental chemicals, even those used in the past, may affect the health of the current generation of reproductive-age women with regard to a hormonally driven disease.[3]

Another study published by *Environmental Health Perspectives* found that rural men working in close contact with pesticides had a 42% lower sperm count than their urban counterparts. The obvious conclusion from the article was that this was caused by certain pesticides used in farming.[4]

Physicians for Social Responsibility concur that these chemicals endanger male fertility. In fact, globally, sperm counts have been reduced and infertility rates have increased. These physicians refer to The Association of Reproductive Health Professionals who has charted the following trends in reproductive health among men:

- Rising rates of testicular cancer
- Falling sperm counts
- Decrease in testosterone levels
- Fewer male babies being born
- Increases in birth defects

Scientific evidence reveals that these issues are the result of endocrine-disrupting chemicals. Even at very low levels, these chemicals can disrupt normal reproductive processes in adults and, most especially, unborn children, as hormones control infant development in the womb. Foetuses exposed to these hormone-disrupting chemicals can experience malformations of the brain and immune system that can negatively affect them for the duration of their lives.[5]

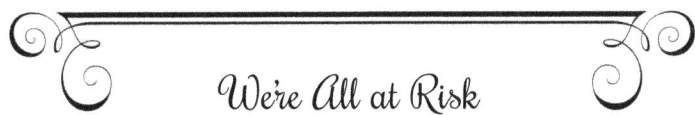

We're All at Risk

Exposure to chemicals weakens and overburdens our immune system, which diminishes our ability to fight off disease. We may not be living in rural agricultural areas, but we are eating the food that has been sprayed and treated with these chemicals. We are therefore also at risk.

ADDED CHEMICALS

Not only are we being amply exposed to all kinds of pesticides through industrial agriculture, but other chemicals are also added to our processed and packaged foods. Detrimental additives are used to either preserve or lengthen the shelf life of these processed products. There is also strong evidence indicating that the combined effects of certain food additives –

including Red dye #3 and # 40, Yellow dye #5 and #6 and Blue dye #1 food colourings – contribute to hyperactivity and learning disabilities in children.[6] Those colourful garnitures on cakes and donuts are actually harmful.

High fructose corn syrup, which spikes our blood sugar levels and raises blood triglycerides, as well as modified cornstarch, are but two GMO corn additives contained in many processed and pre-processed foods. Monosodium glutamate (MSG), hydrolyzed vegetable protein, aspartame and other food enhancers are *excitotoxins*, which are brain neuron disrupters.

EXCITOTOXINS

Excitotoxins are chemical substances added to our food to stimulate the taste buds. These excitotoxins serve no preservative or nutritional purpose but can be hugely harmful. They cause our brain cells to become overly excited. When this happens, these brain cells, which cannot be regenerated, spasm until they die. Dr. Russell Blaylock, author of the book *Excitotoxins: The Taste that Kills*, has researched and written extensively on this subject. He states that consuming foods containing excitotoxins, like MSG and aspartate, has the potential to do irrevocable damage to our brain and nervous system. He cautions that aspartame, a substance found in artificial sweeteners such as NutraSweet®, contains the powerful excitotoxin aspartate and should be avoided at all costs.[7]

> EXCITOTOXINS SERVE NO PRESERVATIVE OR NUTRITIONAL PURPOSE BUT CAN BE HUGELY HARMFUL

What's more, when pregnant women eat processed foods, which contain many food enhancers, these excitotoxins can enter the placenta and damage the brain of unborn children. Dr. Blaylock explains that because of the underdeveloped blood-brain barrier in developing infants and young kids, they are especially prone to damage from exposure to excitotoxins, quite possibly leading to learning disorders, autism, and serious psychological problems.[8]

Excitotoxins also generate extreme levels of free radicals that cause additional cell death. The food industry has been adding MSG to prepared foods since the late 1940's. In one of the Blaylock "Wellness Reports", Dr. Blaylock writes that since the 1980s, Americans have consumed

282,000 metric tonnes of MSG and 800 million pounds of aspartame.[9] In this same report, he states that excitotoxicity has far reaching effects and plays a major role in many life-threatening diseases such as:

- Stroke
- Brain injury
- Brain tumors
- Degenerative brain diseases (Alzheimer's, Parkinson's and Lou Gehrig's disease)
- Meningitis
- Neurological Lyme disease
- Encephalitis
- Schizophrenia
- Depression
- Bipolar disorder
- Addiction behaviours
- Multiple sclerosis

In addition, he states that there is strong evidence that excitotoxins play a central role in autism. He further adds that excitotoxicity also plays a role in a great number of diseases other than brain disorders including the following:

- Diabetes
- Glaucoma
- Migraine headaches
- Metabolic Syndrome
- Atherosclerosis
- Menstrual disorders
- Infertility
- Asthma
- Immune problems
- Cancer

In his book, Blaylock provides a partial list of the most common names for disguised MSG. He reminds us that the powerful excitotoxins aspartate and L-cysteine are more commonly added to foods than we might think. What's more, according to FDA rules, they require no labelling.

Be aware that even though you may not see "MSG" listed in the ingredients, MSG or other excitotoxins may still exist in food products. They may be disguised as one of the ingredients mentioned in the following chart. MSG is present in most prepared foods; this includes restaurant foods – even in restaurants that claim that they add no MSG. Many of the foods they receive from their food suppliers may already contain MSG or other ingredients that camouflage MSG.[10]

ADDITIVES THAT ALWAYS CONTAIN MSG	ADDITIVES THAT FREQUENTLY CONTAIN MSG	ADDITIVES THAT MAY CONTAIN MSG OR OTHER EXCITOTOXINS
• Monosodium glutamate • Hydrolyzed vegetable protein • Hydrolyzed protein • Hydrolyzed plant protein • Plant protein extract • Sodium caseinate • Calcium caseinate • Yeast extract • Textured protein • Autolyzed yeast • Hydrolyzed oat flour	• Malt extract • Malt flavouring • Bouillon • Broth • Stock • Flavouring • Natural flavouring • Natural beef or chicken flavouring • Seasoning • Spices	• Carrageenan • Enzymes • Soy protein concentrate • Soy protein isolate • Whey protein concentrate (Protease enzymes of various sources can release excitotoxic amino acids from food proteins.)

These are but a few of the harmful additives found in processed foods. What can you do to avoid these harmful substances? Reduce consumption of processed foods! When buying groceries, shop on the outside aisle of your food market. Many of these toxic food additives are found in food products that are located in the middle aisles. When buying packaged and canned foods make sure to read your labels carefully.

Many new food products are being added to our supermarket shelves every year. These attractively packaged food products are often full of low-nutrient foods loaded with preservatives, colorants, trans fats, sugar, and excitotoxins, which are all additives that contribute to the toxic overload in our body. We look at the labels to figure out caloric intake, but we don't realize that it's the addition of preservatives and other chemicals, as well as the lack of vital micronutrients, that keep us from being healthy and disease-free. As you are beginning to see, we are being exposed to many more toxins than we realize.

PRESCRIPTION DRUGS

Drug intake of any kind is not something to take lightly. Even seemingly inconsequential, over-the-counter drugs such as painkillers, when taken in large doses, can be responsible for serious liver damage, acute liver failure and even death.[11]

All drugs, whether it be prescription, over-the-counter or recreational drugs, must pass through our liver to be broken down into smaller elements. This added workload not only impairs the many other important liver functions, but can also cause liver damage, starting with inflammation and even leading to cancer. Be reminded that all drugs have some kind of side effect.

Dr. Ray Strand in his book *Death by Prescription* states that all drugs are inherently dangerous. He sites that there are over 100,000 deaths per year in the U.S. from side effects of medication and 80,000 more due to prescription errors or in not respecting the proper dosage.[12] He also adds that thousands of people die each year for taking drugs that treat only minor health problems. This is distressing. Pharmaceutical advertisements have conditioned us to run to the drug store for almost every trivial malaise we encounter. However, what we may not be aware of is that there are many healthy alternatives to ease, reduce and even eliminate minor annoyances like headaches, cold symptoms and cramps. One reason we may not be aware of these alternatives is because we are so accustomed to running to the pharmacy to look for quick, easy solutions, convinced that nothing but medication will relieve our symptoms.

We confide in doctors who normally have not studied holistic remedies and so are not equipped to treat nor guide us with this practice. For example, doctors often prescribe medication to reduce high blood sugar.

Alternatively, changing our diets and lifestyles often gets to the root cause of such ailments. In many cases incorporating these lifestyle changes may actually resolve blood sugar issues. Medical doctors may also prescribe statin drugs to reduce cholesterol, while changing our diet and reducing stress is often just as efficient but has no dangerous side effects. Obviously, our medical system is well designed to respond to emergency intervention and diagnostics, but it is not adapted to personalized, preventive holistic care.

> **WE ARE BEING EXPOSED TO MANY MORE TOXINS THAN WE THINK**

Questioning, researching and evaluating the pros and cons of all drug consumption – even prescribed medication – before hastily consuming them is crucial. Being open to seeking alternative methods and finding the right support is one way for you to start taking responsibility for your health. I assure you, being proactive with your health today can greatly reduce invasive medical intervention later on.

PERFUMES AND PERSONAL CARE PRODUCTS

We have looked at some of the hazardous substances that we ingest through our mouths, often not consciously aware of the damage this brings to our bodies. Now, let's look at the substances that we breathe into our lungs and the harmful preservatives and other toxins that we absorb through our skin. These synthetic scents and preservatives intoxicate our system. They disrupt our hormones, contribute to a compromised immune system and possibly lead to such serious diseases as cancer.

Remember

Most perfumes that we use to make us smell and feel so good are actually detrimental to our health. They are concocted in laboratories with most probably some natural products. However, a large percentage of these commercial fragrances are made from harmful synthetic compounds derived from petrochemicals.

It's remarkable to note the amount of toxic odours we inhale throughout the day. Nice-smelling perfumes are more obvious to detect, but think of the deodorant or antiperspirant you put on every day. Antiperspirants are even more harmful than deodorants because they contain dangerous aluminum inhibitors that block the natural flow of toxins from exiting your body.

Then there are the shampoos, the facial, hand and body creams, all chemically perfumed, that we lavishly slather on our body. These personal care products contain not only chemical scents, but also phthalates and preservatives such as parabens. Phthalates, which are plasticizer chemicals that make personal-care products easier to handle and apply, like in nail polish and hair sprays, are suspected endocrine disruptors. The male reproductive system appears to be more sensitive to these chemicals.[13] Parabens are used to help stop the growth of harmful bacteria and mold, however they have been linked to hormone disruption and breast cancer. There are often many other harmful ingredients in personal care products. Visit safecosmetics.org to find out what chemicals are in yours.

Additionally, some children's bedrooms are furnished with "plug-ins", a chemical air freshener plugged into the electrical socket, releasing a constant toxic scent all day and all night. These chemical perfumes are compromising the health of everyone exposed to it. An equally irritating toxic exposure, in my opinion, is the bathroom sprays used to mask toilet odours. These are potent sprays, which is perhaps why they are so effective. However, is making our homes smell "good" really worth the exposure?

Alternatives to using harmful deodorizing sprays might be simply opening up a window. Or, if there isn't one available, try lighting a small beeswax or other non-toxic candle to burn up any undesirable lingering odour. An essential oil diffuser is also an excellent option as it releases a healthy, natural aroma. Not only do these natural oils not give off toxic chemicals (providing they are organic), but they also have many wonderful therapeutic benefits. Lavender, for example, reduces anxiety and emotional stress, improves your sleep, and it also helps heal burns and wounds. Lemon essential oil helps uplift your mood, and because of its antiviral and antibacterial properties, is great for cleaning. Essential oils are very potent and so a small drop goes a long way.

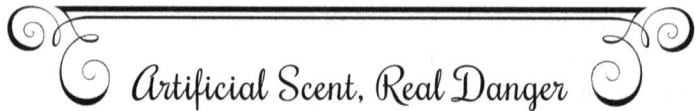

Artificial Scent, Real Danger

Artificial scents are among the top substances known to trigger allergies and asthma attacks. They contain chemicals that are detrimental to our health. We heartily take in deep whiffs of these dangerously camouflaged toxins without even thinking about it.

Many of these toxic ingredients are not listed on labels because manufacturers are allowed to group them into a category called "fragrance" through a governmental loophole. Consequently, they are under no obligation to disclose their "secret formula". However, dozens of toxic chemicals may lurk behind the ingredients listed as "fragrance" on our scented products. According to a report released by The Campaign for Safe Cosmetics, some 38 unlisted chemicals go into top name-brand perfumes, such as Calvin Klein®, Chanel® and Old Spice®, to name a few.[14]

These toxic chemical products – along with other household products, such as lotions, sprays and detergents – contain volatile ingredients that can react dangerously with the already compromised air in our homes. This mix can potentially create secondary air pollutants, such as formaldehyde* and ultrafine particles*, causing all kinds of respiratory ailments.[15]

The Environmental Working Group, a non-profit, non-partisan organization dedicated to protecting human health and the environment, reported the following:

An analysis of the chemical contents of products reveals that the innocuous-looking "fragrance" often contains chemicals linked to negative health effects. Phthalates, used to make fragrances last longer, are associated [with] damage to the male reproductive system, and artificial musks accumulate in our body and can be found in breast milk. Some artificial musks are even linked to cancer.[16]

To avoid fragrances and their associated health risks, look for fragrance-free products. Be careful to avoid labels that use the word "unscented,"

---

* A health-compromising gaseous substance which is a known carcinogen.
** Ambient particles that are small enough to enter directly into the lung cavities.

however, as there may be another chemical fragrance added to cover up or neutralize the product's original odour.

The presence of menacing toxins in personal care products goes on and on. Think about hair dyes, makeup and anti-aging wrinkle creams that we put on our face ... and powder on our eyes ... and lipstick on our lips ... and so on, and so on. These products all contain harmful chemicals. Many lipsticks, for example, contain lead. When we add everything up, these chemicals can have an enormous negative impact on the state of our health. An article in *The Globe and Mail* cites The Campaign for Safe Cosmetics in stating that the average person is exposed to 126 toxic chemicals from personal care products alone, per day.[17] I'm not saying that we must stop all use of these products, but we must diminish their use if we want to stay on the road to optimal health.

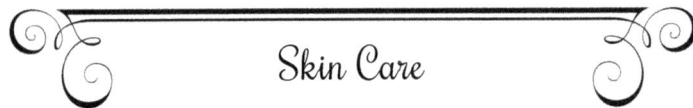

Skin Care

Your skin is the largest organ of your body. The surface is substantial and able to absorb a great amount of substances. Be mindful not only of what you put in your body but also what you put on it. There are more and more preservative-free and toxin-free personal care products available on the market today – opt for these instead.

HAND SANITIZERS AND ANTIBACTERIAL SOAPS AND WASHES

Personal hygiene and cleanliness is very important for the prevention or spreading of contagious diseases. In fact, regularly washing our hands with soap and water for at least 20 seconds effectively destroys bacteria and viruses. However, some think we need even more protection and have turned to the regular and repeated use of hand sanitizers. Many hand sanitizers contain antibacterial ingredients such as triclosan. This harmful chemical can also be found added to clothes, furniture and toys. It leads to hormonal disruptions in animals, can negatively affect human immune function and can also contribute to the development of anti-biotic resistant bacteria.[18] This resistance develops through a process called "cross resistance". The bacteria adapts and grows stronger and becomes more resistant to the effects of other antibiotics, even though they have not been exposed to them directly, leading to the rise of so called "super bugs".

Some people are concerned about hygiene to an extreme extent. However, the problem with using antibacterial agents such as triclosan is that it kills bad as well as beneficial bacteria. We shouldn't strive to live in a totally germ-free environment. A little bit of bad bacteria is not to be feared as their presence actually helps to develop our immune system. No need to be overly cautious for toddlers and young children as they are equipped with a fully working immune-enhancing thymus gland which is at its peak performance in their younger age. Nature has many wonderful ways of protecting us!

In fact, keeping young children in an overly clean or sterilized environment can contribute to a malfunctioning immune system later on in life. This is because it was not properly stimulated when growing up. Once children reach puberty – when they have hopefully developed the notion and discipline of proper hygiene – the thymus starts to slowly shrink and its functions gradually decrease.

Hand sanitizers may have their place, providing they are not overused. When needed, choose the alcohol-based hand sanitizers and make sure they are fragrance free, as fragrances contain phthalates, which we now know cause damage to the reproductive system, especially to unborn baby boys.[19] Use them only when necessary as these types of alcohol are neurotoxic and can be absorbed through the skin. Avoid using them if your hands are cracked as this can allow the toxic chemicals found in the hand sanitizer itself to penetrate the skin easier. Basically, washing with regular soap and water is almost always a better choice.

HOME CLEANING PRODUCTS

Another vast area of exposure to toxic substances comes from all the household products we use to clean our homes, kitchens, bathrooms and cars. Think also about your laundry. Detergents and especially synthetic fabric softeners contain many dangerous chemical perfumes. You can decrease your toxic load simply by substituting these products with more natural ones. For instance, use vinegar in your rinse cycle to remove any odours. We need to get used to linking "no smell" with "healthy smell." Otherwise, you can always apply a few drops of essential oils on your skin to add healthy and pleasant natural scents. Know that there now exist many non-toxic, biologically friendly alternatives for our many cleaning necessities.

The clothes that we bring back from the dry cleaners are also loaded with harmful chemicals. Hang them outside to dissipate the chemical odours before bringing them into your home. New clothes that you bring home from a shopping spree are also covered with chemicals used to prevent mildew and to keep them from wrinkling. Clothing comes in direct contact with your skin, therefore these toxins get absorbed through your pores. Wash all new clothes before you wear them.

"NO SMELL" EQUALS "HEALTHY SMELL"

BISPHENOL A

If we take a short visit to the kitchen and see what our foods are stored in, we will probably encounter a lot of plastic containers. Certain plastic containers leach bisphenol A (BPA) into our foods. Bisphenol A is a toxic substance that mimics the hormone oestrogen. This oestrogen imitation disturbs men's, women's and children's hormonal systems and can lead to cancer. Glass bottles and glass or metal containers are the safest storage containers because they do not contain BPA. Note that there are some plastics that are BPA free.

Canned foods and beverage receptacles lined with plastic coating can also leach BPAs. Following is an excerpt from an article on *The Globe and Mail* website explaining the dangers of BPAs:

Scientists have warned that BPA could interfere with numerous biological processes because its structure resembles the hormone estrogen. It has been shown to interfere with reproductive development in animals and it has been linked to cardiovascular disease, diabetes and obesity in humans. Aside from cans, it's also used to make some hard, clear plastics, dentistry composites and sealants and some cash register receipts.[20]

Many plastic water bottles are advertised as BPA free, but some may contain Bisphenol S (BPS), a similar substance that is equally as toxic if not more. Therefore, you would be best served by avoiding plastics near your food and water wherever possible, unless of course you are confident of the source.

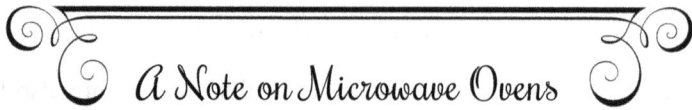

A Note on Microwave Ovens

Please, if you insist on using a microwave to warm your foods, and I hope it is very occasionally, do not warm it in a plastic receptacle or worse yet Styrofoam®. The heat from the microwave causes BPA and other toxins to leach out from the plastic or Styrofoam® into your food!

NON-STICK COOKWARE

Although convenient and easy-to-clean, non-stick cookware is very toxic when exposed to high heat. The toxic off-gassing has been known to kill canaries and other pet birds in the nearby surroundings of heated Teflon® cookware. Toxins are released when the pan is exposed to high heat – sometimes you can even see the pan smoking; this is very carcinogenic. We breathe in these fumes while nonchalantly stir-frying our fresh vegetables. If these fumes kill birds, they will also harm us.[21] Additionally, with use, the non-stick adhesive layer begins to deteriorate, and we actually end up eating small portions of these non-stick substances. Instead of using Teflon® coated pots and pans, use stainless steel, glass or cast iron cookware. These do not produce toxic gases. Additionally, avoid aluminum cookware, as it is a toxin that harms our respiratory, musculoskeletal and nervous systems. In fact, abnormal levels of aluminum have been found in the brains of people with Alzheimer's disease.[22]

A WORD ON COOKING WITH HIGH HEAT

Cooking meats like beef, chicken, fish and pork with high heat, especially over 300 degrees F (150 degrees C) creates a cancer causing substance. The elements necessary to create this substance called heterocyclic amines (HCA's) are protein, creatinine and sugar, all of which are found in the muscle of these meats. HCAs are mutagenic, which means they can alter our DNA.[23]

The flames coming from the drippings of fats and juices from meats cooked over an open fire or a barbeque produce another cancer causing substance, called polycyclic aromatic hydrocarbon (PAH), which then sticks to the surface of the meat.[24] Therefore, keep barbeques and other dry heat cooking for special occasions only.

Acrylamide is yet another toxic substance created when high carbohydrate/low protein foods are cooked at high temperatures of 248 F (120 C) and above. Potato chips and commercial breakfast cereals, pretzels and roasted coffee beans are some examples of acrylamide containing foods.

Another unhealthy chemical reaction called Advanced Glycation End products (AGEs) is generated when proteins or fats along with sugars are heated above 248 F (120 C). The proteins and fats in meats makes them also very prone to the formation of AGEs, especially when cooking with high, dry heat. Marinating uncooked meats in an acidic medium such as vinegar or lemon juice helps reduce AGE production during the cooking process.[25]

A diet high in sugar, such as candy, cookies, cakes, pastries, soft drinks and other processed and pre-packaged foods, also contributes to higher AGE consumption. AGEs irritate cells, cause tissue damage, inflammation and premature aging. The more sugar you eat – not dismissing the hidden sugars added in processed foods – the higher the production of AGEs. High AGE consumption is known to increase the risk for diseases like diabetes, Alzheimer's disease and heart disease.[26] It can also compromise the maintenance of collagen in our bodies. The extra sugar molecules bind with the collagen and elastin proteins, causing wrinkles and loss of elasticity. Eating lots of raw, or lightly steamed vegetables and low-sugar fruit (such as berries) not only prevents us from filling up on foods high in AGEs, but may also reduce the new formation of AGEs. This is perhaps due to the higher water content and higher level of antioxidants and vitamins found in fruits and vegetables.

Finally, when cooking foods, all foods should be cooked slowly and with low heat. Cooking in water such as poaching, steaming, boiling, or in a slow cooker, creates very few of the afore mentioned toxic substances, as opposed to dry heat cooking such as barbecue, grilling, pan frying, broiling and even baking at high temperatures. In addition, cooking with low heat retains more vitamin and mineral content and allows for easier digestion and assimilation of our meals. Incidentally, if you have to boil certain vegetables instead of steaming them, keep the nutrient filled water for a healthy base when making your homemade soups or sauces.

WATER

Finally, let's look at municipal, treated water. Treated tap water exposes us to many chemicals including chlorine and – depending on where you live – fluoride, both of which contribute to toxic overload in our body. According to the Canadian Cancer Society (CCS), even though chlorine disinfects the water and makes it safe for us to drink, when it interacts with organic matter, such as dead leaves and soil present in the water prior to treatment, it forms new chemicals that remain in the water. These chlorination by-products can increase the risk of cancer. CCS also mentions that these by-products are:

...possible causes of cancer and that the most common chlorination by-products called trihalomethanes (THMs) and haloacetic acids (HAAs), can cause cancer in laboratory animals. Many studies have shown that long-term exposure slightly increases the risk of bladder cancer. Other studies have also deduced links to colorectal cancer and these chlorination by-products.[27]

Filtering your drinking water is crucial. Consider investing in a water filter for your home and enjoy the many benefits and conveniences. Connecting a central unit directly to your main water inlet would be the absolute best. If this is not financially possible, you could purchase a water distiller providing you are taking a proven good quality multi-vitamin and multi-mineral supplement, as a water distiller removes most everything out of your water including minerals. You can also add in a small amount of raw, organic apple cider vinegar to your distilled water to bring back some live active nutrients, enzymes and probiotics.

There are other good quality water filters that you can attach directly to your kitchen tap; a reverse osmosis water filter is an excellent option. Make sure you do your research prior to purchase. You may also want to look into a Kangen® water system unit, an innovative water technology which produces ionized alkaline water. It is has been said that drinking alkaline water between meals has many benefits, one being the reduction of acidity in your body. A cost effective option would be the use of a Brita® water pitcher filter. However, the carbon filter that removes the chlorine from your drinking water is limited in its capacity to eliminate all chemicals and contaminants, and does not remove fluoride. It's a good first step if you are in a city that doesn't fluoridate its drinking water. Remember to periodically change your filters.

Breathing in water vapour while showering and even while swimming also exposes us to these toxins. Installing a showerhead filter can help significantly to remove chlorine and other chemicals from your shower.

FLUORIDE

Fluoride in our water and in our toothpaste is harmful to us. This is a very controversial topic as the American Dental Association (ADA) is in favour of using fluoride for preventing cavities and assures us that it is safe. However, they caution that if you feed your baby primarily powdered infant formula, preparing it using fluoridated water might increase the chance for mild enamel fluorosis. These discoloured spots on teeth are caused by overexposure to fluoride during childhood. To decrease the chance of enamel fluorosis the ADA suggests that mothers either breast feed – as breast milk is low in fluoride – or use a formula mixed with fluoride-free water or water that contains low levels of fluoride. This recommendation seems somewhat contradicting.

Also note that fluoridated toothpastes contain a warning cautioning not to leave young children under the age of six alone to brush their teeth – for fear of swallowing too much fluoride. If swallowing too much fluoride contained in toothpaste damages teeth enamel on teeth that are still forming, could swallowing the fluoride contained in the drinking water or added to our food or drinks also create disturbances in other parts of our body – our bones and our organs, for instance?

An article from the Fluoride Action Network (FAN) states that:

(…) a growing body of evidence reasonably indicates that fluoridated water, in addition to other sources of daily fluoride exposure, can cause or contribute to a range of serious effects, including arthritis, damage to the

developing brain, reduced thyroid function, and possibly osteosarcoma (bone cancer) in adolescent males.[28]

Fluoride is known to displace iodine in our body, an element essential for the proper functioning of the thyroid gland. Lack of iodine causes hypothyroidism, an ever-expanding health ailment.[29] According to another article posted on the FAN website, all active cells require thyroid hormones for proper functioning, therefore if the thyroid gland is dysfunctional this can have an effect on almost every system of the body.[30]

If your city water is fluoridated and you don't want to be exposed to this, you may wish to use a water filter that removes fluoride. If you don't have such a water filter, you can purchase from your local grocery store large jugs of water that have been properly filtered. If they don't have glass jugs available, request them, or at least make sure that the refillable plastic jugs made available to you do not contain PBA or BPS. Additionally, replace your fluoride toothpastes with natural, non-toxic toothpastes. Read all ingredients in packaged food and drinks as some may contain fluoride.

How to Reduce Cavities

Tooth decay is not caused by a lack of fluoride but from a bad diet and improper dental hygiene. Therefore it is not necessary to supplement with fluoride by adding it to toothpaste, water or food. A safer way of reducing cavities is to reduce sugar intake and eat a diet rich in minerals, in addition to brushing your teeth and flossing regularly.

SILVER AMALGAM FILLINGS

Although now proven to be very toxic, silver amalgam fillings are still being used by many dentists. They are even authorized by the government. The danger with these kinds of fillings, is that they contain mercury. Mercury is a poison; it is toxic, even in minute amounts. The ADA (American Dental Association) tries to reassure us by affirming that amalgam fillings are in no way dangerous. However, there are many doctors and specialists who have written on the dangers of mercury poisoning from amalgam fillings. Dr. Myron Wentz, a world-renowned expert in virology and cellular immunology states in his book *A Mouth Full of Poison* that brushing our teeth and chewing our food continually releases mercury vapour from our silver amalgam fillings. This contributes to the cumulative increase of this poison in the tissues of our body, notably in the kidneys and the central nervous system. He further states that exposure to mercury is known to be the initial cause of the following diseases:[31]

- Acrodynia
- Alzheimer's
- Arthritis
- Asthma
- Autism
- Candida
- Developmental defects
- Senile dementia
- Depression
- Liver disorders
- Immune system disorders
- Reproductive system disorders
- Diabetes
- Learning disabilities
- Hormonal dysfunction
- Intestinal dysfunction
- Eczema
- Emphysema
- Metabolic encephalopathy
- Fibromyalgia
- Renal insufficiency
- Cardiovascular disease
- Crohn's disease
- Disease of the thyroid gland
- Parkinson's disease
- Multiple Sclerosis
- Amyotrophic Lateral Sclerosis
- Chronic Fatigue Syndrome

Dr. Wentz advises those who have amalgam fillings to have them replaced for their greater security. He also stresses how crucial it is to understand that you will never find complete health if you have silver amalgam fillings in your mouth continually releasing mercury vapors that are then absorbed in your body.

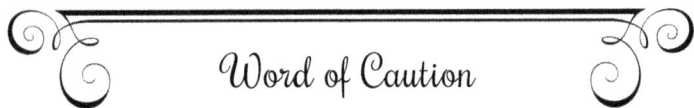

Word of Caution

If you decide to remove your amalgam fillings, please make sure you consult a dentist who takes strict precautionary measures when doing so. If you are pregnant or breast-feeding do not attempt this procedure as the mercury released when removing amalgam fillings can cause harm to babies in utero as well as to the breast-fed child.

The prevalence of autism is on the rise and there may be a direct correlation with mercury poisoning.[32] If you are planning to have children, it would be wise to remove your silver amalgam fillings several months prior to conception. The IAOMT (International Academy of Oral Medicine and Technology) has developed rigorous recommendations for the removal of amalgams called Safe Mercury Amalgam Removal Techniques (SMART). They also host a member's list of dentists who are educated in biological dentistry.[33]

VACCINES

Today, more and more people are beginning to question the efficacy and safety of vaccinations. Babies and young children are receiving many more vaccines with more frequent doses. Are all of these vaccines necessary? Take for instance the Hepatitis B vaccine. It has been added to the child vaccination schedule and administered to most one-day-old US babies to protect them from a disease that is either sexually transmitted or blood born (ex: through IV drug use).[34] Should parents who are not at risk be obligated to subject their newborns to this additional vaccine?

While the number of vaccines has been increasing, it is interesting to note that there has been a substantial increase in learning disabilities, including ADD, ADHD, an increase in asthma, allergies and other autoimmune diseases, as well as an epidemical increase in Autism.[35] Could there possibly be a link between these growing number of disorders, chronic illnesses and vaccinations? Could we be over vaccinating? Could vaccines be toxic? These questions are not something to be taken lightly. The health of today's children is in jeopardy and questions must be asked. New and more vaccinations will most likely continue to be added to the child vaccination schedule. Who is behind this increase of vaccinations? Are they all crucial and necessary? There even exists an adolescent "recommended" immunization schedule.[36] Vaccines that are now being administered to adults are on the increase as well.

What about getting naturally acquired immunity through exposure to infectious diseases? No one likes getting sick, but it is a natural part of life. Our body fights against viruses by creating a fever. Fever is a good thing. It is our body's natural means of killing bacteria and viruses. When doing so it develops its immune response, making it stronger and creating lifelong immunity in the process. As adults, are we becoming dependant on vaccines so we don't have to suffer the effects of having the flu? Or are we accepting a flu vaccine out of fear of going against what doctors are suggesting, or fear of a pandemic outbreak if we don't get vaccinated? Regardless, flu shots are not 100% foolproof.

The CDC (Center for Disease Control) says that, "flu shots vary in effectiveness from season-to-season depending on how well scientists accurately predicted the current season's primary flu strain". They say that the average flu shot is 50-60% effective, *providing* there is a good match between the vaccine and the circulating flu virus. But even so, the benefits may vary. They also mention that it is possible that no benefits from flu vaccinations may be observed.[37]

The best way to prevent sickness from any virus is to have a good working immune system. And that comes from good nutrition, regular exercise and a healthy lifestyle, including the reduction of the number of toxins entering our bodies. Washing your hands with soap and water frequently, as well as coughing or sneezing in the bend of your arm, not your hand, does wonders for protecting yourself as well as those around you. Unless you have a compromised immune system, your body is well equipped to fight for you. Do not let fear scare you into taking any vaccine. Knowledge gives us confidence to make well-thought out and calculated decisions. Please get informed before making yours.

HARMFUL INGREDIENTS

Do you really know what is in a flu vaccine? In actual fact, all vaccines contain toxic ingredients. Increased vaccinations are resulting in an increased accumulation of toxins in our bodies, as well as those of our children. Vaccines contain dangerous ingredients such as: mercury (from thimerosal), formaldehyde (a human carcinogen), magnesium sulfate (frequently used as a fertilizer), monosodium glutamate (MSG), and aluminum (a neurotoxin) just to name a few.[38] These poisons, once injected into our body, compromise our immune systems.

Even pregnant moms are now recommended to take the flu shot, "in order to protect themselves and their baby". They are told that the protection the vaccinated mother gets while pregnant may transfer across the placenta and stay with their baby for a short time after birth.[39] If the protection from the virus crosses the placenta, then the toxins in these vaccines, like mercury and aluminum for instance, will also cross the placenta. These are neurotoxic elements and are dangerous for a baby's neurological development. How can the government justify recommending pregnant women to limit their consumption of certain types of fish, because if "eaten too frequently, [it] could result in exposure to an unacceptable amount of mercury" – while encouraging them to get a flu vaccine that contains even higher levels of unacceptable amounts of mercury?[40]

We follow governmental and medical directives, doing what is recommended, never questioning if this is safe for us and our children, assuming that they have our safety in mind. Could it be possible that the pharmaceutical industry's focus on corporate profit-increase bring direction and influence regarding the increased production and marketing of vaccines? We can no longer continue to blindly accept what they propose. We have the right to ask questions. We have heard one side of the story, maintaining that vaccines are safe and necessary. It may be wise to hear the other side of the story.

Take the time to view "VaxXed Tour" or "VaxXed Stories" on YouTube to hear real stories about moms (and dads) and their challenges regarding vaccinations and their children. Part of taking responsibility for our health involves researching and becoming informed. There is an explosion of information available for us today. Please do your research. The on-line documentary called *Silent Epidemic, The Untold Story of Vaccines*, one of many on-line documentaries, is a great place to start to get some information in order to get another perspective on this issue. Being a member of the online Vaccine Research Library can give you access to articles posted on the most recent medical literature.

I urge you, especially if you are parents to small children, to get informed. Look into alternative scheduling. Be aware of the potential risks of multiple dose vaccinations. Look at each vaccine, find out what is in it, and know what illness it is treating. Know your individual child's risk, both of getting the disease and potential harm from the vaccine. Find out how natural lifelong immunity is built into the body. Verify if vaccine-induced herd immunity* really exists.[41]

---

* also called community immunity.

Regardless of your choices or convictions regarding this controversial subject, boosting your immune system is imperative. The best health heritage you can give your baby is to boost your own immune system before getting pregnant. If you are a pregnant mom, know that what you eat or don't eat can either be contributing to or taking away from your baby's future immune system. In addition, having a natural birth permits babies to receive additional protective bacteria from the birth canal that helps kick start their immune system. Having a C-section does not enable this. Although giving birth naturally is best, life does not always go as planned and at times, certain uncontrollable situations may impose a C-section. Breastfeeding also helps contribute to your baby's immune system. Once again, there are some women who can't breastfeed their baby for various reasons. If you find yourself in any one of these situations, please do not feel guilty. You'll just have to work a little harder to strengthen your baby's immunity by applying advice received from qualified people.

It is your fundamental right as well as your responsibility to make educated, well informed decisions both for your own body and that of your child's. Be wise and open to learning and begin to apply what you learn.

ELECTROMAGNETIC FIELDS

Electromagnetic fields (EMF) are emitted from electrical devices and power lines. They are also radiated from the use of cordless phones, cell phones, mobile antennas, broadcast towers, smart meters, electrical alarm systems, Wi-Fi, microwaves, airplane travel and more.

Many assert that there is presently no conclusive evidence that proves any serious negative impacts of EMF radiation on human health. However, even though exposure to one source of EMF may seem to be insignificant, there is growing concern that the compounded effect of multiple exposure, as well as length and strength of exposure, may be a serious health risk especially experienced by those who are electro-sensitive. Infants and small children may be even more at risk.

Specialists consider exposure to intense EMF to interfere with our body's own bioelectrical signals. This interference may negatively affect our inner bodies' communication systems that regulate different processes such as our sleep cycles, stress levels, immunity, heart rate and may even affect our DNA.[42] So if you want to be safe, train yourself to identify sources of invisible EMF emanating around you and take proactive measures to reduce your exposure whenever you can. For instance, you can turn your WIFI off at night and make sure your cell phones are nowhere near your bed while you are sleeping.

EMF emission strength decreases with distance. For example, there is a radical decline of intensity when distancing yourself anywhere from 10 to 15 inches (30 to 40 cm) from your cell phone, or 3 to 5 feet (1 to 1.5 metres) from you cordless phone base, and 6 feet (approximately 2 metres) from your microwave oven.[43] Another way of being proactive, is to put your cell phone on speaker phone when you can, spend less time on cordless phones and refrain from resting your lap top on your lap. Consider keeping your portable phone base a good distance away from where you spend most of your time, at least 6 feet; it is constantly emanating EMF waves regardless of whether you are on the phone or not. Women should avoid resting their cell phone on their chest, or worse yet on their belly when they are pregnant; it may well interfere with the heart's bio-electrical signals. Walking barefoot on the grass for 15 minutes is a good way of discharging electromagnetic energy from your body. This is also very beneficial after an airplane flight!

BE EMPOWERED

I know that we have covered a lot of information on the toxins that surround us and how they negatively affect our health. I realize that this can be overwhelming and perhaps discouraging for some. However, my goal is to empower you. The power of awareness and understanding leads us to be able to make healthy choices. Being ignorant of what contributes to illness prevents us from making those necessary beneficial changes. With knowledge and understanding we can better face what is before us and make some healthy adjustments before damaging consequences set in. Be encouraged. With the help of God and with support from those well equipped to assist you, you can counter, even reverse, debilitating symptoms and disease.

Nothing in life is to be feared, it is only to be understood.
Now is the time to understand more, so that we may fear less.

~ Marie Curie

So please be brave, fearless and feel empowered as you continue learning what is necessary to get great health. There is one more subject I would like to touch on which raises awareness to a different kind of toxin, one that we may be producing inside of our own bodies.

NEGATIVE EMOTIONS

Negative emotions leading to stress are big contributors to disease. We often don't realize how much stress affects us. Conflicts in our personal and work relationships can trigger detrimental negative emotions, such as anger, bitterness, rejection and resentment. These emotions can increase blood pressure and release harmful chemicals in the body. Long-term stress can exhaust our adrenal glands, which in turn can cause bouts of low blood pressure and extreme fatigue. If these emotions are not addressed and resolved, over time they can actually be the foundation for some serious diseases, including cancer.

The California Department of Health Services conducted a joint-study of 847 women with breast cancer over a nine year period and found that those who repressed emotions like anger and grief were four times more likely to die from cancer.[44] This study also cites Dr. W. Douglas Brodie, founder of the Reno Integrative Medical Center in Nevada. He stated:

The cancer-susceptible individual harbors long-suppressed toxic emotions, such as anger, resentment and / or hostility. They typically internalize such emotions and have great difficulty expressing them.[45]

It seems that so many of our friends and family are randomly being hit with cancer, and we, bewildered, conclude that this has struck out of nowhere. In fact, un-dealt with negative emotions are very destructive and are many times at the root of these cancers. We must help our close ones find a qualified person in whom they can confide in order to help guide them in identifying and releasing these toxic emotions before they destroy their bodies.

SELF-EXAMINATION

If you really want to live a healthy life, you must take a serious look at all areas of stress in your life. Start asking yourself some hard questions regarding your subconscious motivations as well as your ability to set and maintain healthy boundaries. Sometimes it's easier to sweep irritations under the carpet, or succumb to constant demands put upon you because you don't want to disappoint or be rejected. Or you may simply choose, consciously or unconsciously, to shut down emotionally or to remain in denial. This still creates stress, but on an unconscious level.

THE STRESS HORMONES

Stress activates the fight-or-flight system in our body by producing the stress hormones adrenaline and cortisol. Adrenaline produces a surge of energy in us. It's excellent for getting us out of physical danger. We have heard of superhuman feats, like a woman lifting a car that had her child pinned under the wheel. That's the power of adrenaline. It's an energy boost that can literally save us from danger.

The problem is that adrenaline is activated by any kind of stress. So if you are very upset with someone, or if you are required to produce a report before the end of the week, for example, and you know that you may not have enough time to complete it, you may inadvertently be producing too much adrenaline. The dilemma is that this adrenaline that gives you extra energy, is mostly produced to give your muscles a physical boost. When you are angry or stressed behind your desk at work, you usually don't engage in a physical response like running for your life or lifting super heavy objects to save someone. Often times stress that triggers adrenaline to help you fight or flee can do you great harm when you remain sedentary. A little bit of adrenaline or cortisol is good – actually, cortisol helps you get out of bed in the morning. However, the over-production of these hormones, if carried on for long periods of time, can contribute to a weakened and diseased body.

> ADRENALINE IS AN ENERGY BOOST THAT CAN SAVE YOU FROM DANGER

When the body is focused on getting us out of a perceived dangerous situation or any other stressful dilemma, the production of stress hormones activates the sympathetic nervous system, which is in charge of increased muscle energy production. It also causes more rapid breathing and dilates the pupils so that we can be more focused and capture more detail. All energy that the body deems not important or appropriate to meet the demands of the present perceived emergency is put on hold. When this happens, the parasympathetic nervous system is automatically turned down as the two systems cannot run at full speed simultaneously. That means activities controlled by the parasympathetic nervous system – digestion, reproduction, rest, restoration – are severely diminished. Because cortisol inhibits digestion, the chronic activation of our sympathetic nervous system impairs proper assimilation and absorption of our food. Not only does long-term stress cause inflammation through the chronic over-production of cortisol, it also affects our body's ability to nourish and regenerate itself effectively.

IN CONCLUSION

As you can see there is usually not one specific thing that causes our bodies to break down and succumb to disease, but rather an accumulation of various factors. The more aware we are, the more informed, positive choices we can make, the greater possibility we have of creating a resilient body and mind.

I want to congratulate you for having made it through a substantial amount of sobering information thus far. You are now hopefully more aware and better equipped to start taking an active role in managing your health.

SUMMARY

- **There are toxins all around us.** There are indeed quite a few aspects of everyday living that can contribute to damaging chemicals invading our body. When added altogether, these assaults may insidiously be contributing to the gradual breakdown of a person's health. We have not necessarily been alerted to the dangers of all of these harmful additives in our food, as well as chemicals in our home and work environment.

- **When our cells are suffocating in an oxygen-sparse environment and bathing in toxic waste, they simply are not able to function effectively.** Toxins will keep accumulating inside our body if we continue living and doing the same things that got us toxic in the first place. However, once we understand and are aware of these dangers there are many simple, easy things that we can do to alleviate these negative repercussions. As we gradually incorporate and make small adjustments, we can gain back our health.

- **Chemicals and additives are not the only things negatively impacting our health.** Negative emotions and stress contribute to the breaking down of our immune system. In most cases we don't have immediate symptoms of living a stressful life. We often don't make the connection of cause and effect, and the dangers of exposure go under the radar.

- **The gradual accumulation of all different kinds of toxins inside our body and their negative effects is like the frog being tricked by jumping into the kettle of cold water, slowly increasing in temperature, until finally it dies by boiling to death.** It happened so gradually that the frog didn't realize how hot the water got and didn't even have the reflex to jump out.

- **We can do something about this!** As we become more aware of these dangers we can begin to consciously guard ourselves from their negative effects. Awareness and understanding brings new hope.

In the next chapter, we discover the amazing detoxifying power of our body.

CHAPTER THREE

Toxic overload is a powerful contributor to poor health and a forerunner of so many diseases. The good news is that the body is equipped with several detoxifying systems that help purge these toxins. We have four organs that push toxins outside of our body, as well as two other very important inner assistants, our liver and our lymph, that greatly contribute to the detoxifying process. We will look at each one individually

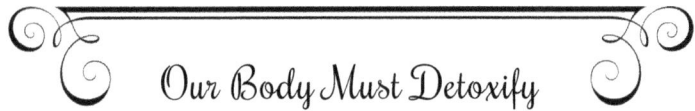

It's critical to understand that the accumulation of residues and toxins in our body weakens it and contributes to its diseased state. Our body has to detoxify. Failure to do so will produce an environment conducive to the development of disease.

To help us better understand this detoxification process, let's go back to the woodstove analogy in chapter 1. Just imagine if that woodstove is in constant operation but never gets cleaned out. The ashes would get so built up that there would be no more room for the fire to burn. No more fire, no more heat (energy).

Although the functioning of our metabolism and digestion is a bit more complicated than the workings of a woodstove, the metaphor here helps us understand that too many toxins in our body, along with lack of oxygen, prevents our cells from working properly. When there is toxic build-up, we feel sluggish and rundown. This becomes a vicious cycle, because we don't have enough oxygen—coming either from clean water, raw fruits and vegetables or from fresh air—to fan the flame and thus revitalize the body. We lack energy and vitality. It's in these times that we can easily get sick. Or worse yet, if this situation becomes chronic, we can end up with a debilitating illness.

THE BOWELS

If we let inappropriate substances go down our household drains, we usually end up with blocked pipes. Ever try flushing a toilet that is already plugged? Not a nice scene. If plugged pipes are not attended to, you can imagine what a cesspool of bacteria this would create. This sewage would begin to seep into the house. The same goes for the body. If we don't evacuate our feces regularly, then the inside of our intestinal track becomes a breeding ground for many bacteria and microbes. When looking at your own kitchen trash or any city park garbage can, you will agree that bacteria and microbes grow where there is garbage. The same holds true inside our body. Toxic wastes that are not regularly expelled from the body cause bad bacteria and microbes to proliferate.

LEAKY GUT SYNDROME

When the colon is exposed to irritating factors, the gut lining increases its permeability. This is called "leaky gut syndrome". That's when undigested food particles, as well as other toxins or bacteria present in our colon, pass through our compromised intestinal wall into our blood stream. This causes allergies, inflammation and other autoimmune conditions. Some contributing factors that lead to leaky gut are: certain inflammatory foods, such as wheat, refined carbs, dairy and sugar; medications such as antibiotics, antacids etc.; and infections such as candida and other bacterial overgrowth.

A Healthy Colon

Our small intestine, which is approximately 20-feet long, is where most of our nutrients are absorbed. Our large intestine or colon, which is approximately 5 feet long, houses many healthy, beneficial bacteria, which also aids in the absorption of certain nutrients. The colon, represented by the plumbing in our analogy, evacuates the toxic fecal matter from our body. It's of utmost importance to have good working bowels. It is well known in the world of alternative medicine that the health of the colon determines the health of the whole body.

Many people don't have regular bowel movements. Some medical doctors seem to think this is okay. They think that it's even normal for some people to have a bowel movement once a week. I have even heard of some having a bowel movement once every two weeks! Many believe that as long as their frequency is consistent – whether it be once a week or once a day – they have no reason to be concerned. These people simply interpret this as an indicator of individual metabolism. Be careful of reaching such a conclusion, it can be perilous.

If two people eat the same meal, they will have the same amount of roughage and refuse remaining from that meal. All of this waste needs to be eliminated regardless of your rate of metabolism. If it is not, having it hanging around in the body for too long will cause putrefaction and create a fertile breeding ground for bacteria, worms and other parasites. Long-term accumulation of this refuse results in hardened fecal waste matter that gets glued to our intestinal wall. This build-up can be one of the reasons why our bellies get distended and a bit harder as the years go by. These old accumulated dehydrated feces combined with latent sticky mucous is also known as mucoid plaque. The elimination of this accumulation of plaque can be dislodged using special herbs along with medicinal fibre.

> **TOXIC MATERIAL HANGING AROUND IN THE BODY FOR TOO LONG IS NOT HEALTHY**

Normally, for every meal we eat, we should have an equal number of bowel movements. I'm sure you must be surprised. Nowadays, I think few people have a bowel movement per meal, but they should. Ideally, after we eat a meal, the small intestine uptakes the molecules of vitamins, minerals, fats and other essential nutrients that will be used to nourish the cells of our body. The rest of the food substances that have not been digested or absorbed, including the fibre, continue down to the large intestine. After the fermentation process and further absorption of certain nutrients, the body will then absorb the water it needs, leaving the undesired feces (waste material) to be evacuated, ideally in approximately 12 to 18 hours.[1]

There should be a daily evacuation of the waste material of each meal. However we won't evacuate each meal right after its consumption. For example, an optimal elimination process could be one bowel movement in the morning, from the previous day's lunch, another some other time during the day from the previous day's supper and one in the evening before retiring for the night from that day's breakfast. When this constant elimination does not happen, we begin to overload our body with residual toxic waste material. As we have mentioned before, this will cause unforeseen problems down the line.

Your bowel movements can tell you a lot about how you eat. They should not be foul smelling, as this would indicate putrefaction. This happens when fecal matter ferments after remaining inside your body for too long, or because of the improper balance between good and bad bacteria. Stools should not be hard nor sticky. Ideally, you should rather quickly dispense of your stool and need very little toilet paper afterwards. If you need a lot of toilet paper, this indicates that your diet is unbalanced and probably lacking in fibre. If your stool sinks quickly to the bottom of the toilet, this also could indicate a lack of fibre as well as dehydration issues. Having any type of problem with this detoxifying organ creates a challenge as your body will be working overtime to try to compensate for this system being blocked up.

What you need to keep in mind is that backed up sewage inside your body can cause many devastating conditions over time.

COLONIC IRRIGATION

Years ago, shortly after the birth of my first child, and soon after I began seeing my first alternative health care practitioner – a bio-nutritionist – I was exposed to my first colonic irrigation. This technique uses a tube to inject water into the colon via the rectum for the removal of accumulated debris. I was so plugged up that I literally blocked the machine. It was not a very positive experience for me and would be the last one for a very long time before it would become an important part of my health detoxifying regime.

Because I chose to no longer do colonic irrigations, my bio-nutritionist urged me to at least buy myself an enema bag and administer one myself at home. So I tried it. I was aghast when I found out that the little white rice particles in the toilet were not white rice at all, but rather tiny maggot-like parasites that were living off of the debris in my intestine! There was more than a cup full! It was the creepiest feeling I have ever had.

I know that this is gross, but I tell you this so that you can understand that a congested colon is a breeding place for all kinds of parasites and bacteria. I am totally convinced that if I had not encountered this bio-nutritionist, who put me on the right path to regaining my health, I would have developed some kind of debilitating degenerative disease. My body was in a very toxic state.

You see, my colon was so full of detritus, which acted as a great host for parasites, that every time I ate a lot of sweets I actually fed these little varmints. The toxins they excreted weakened my immune system. My longstanding processed carbohydrate and sugar addiction also contributed to the production of tons of mucous. All of this was loading down my lymphatic system, a detoxification system of utmost importance on which we will elaborate later. Bacteria were free to proliferate in my body causing me to have numerous throat infections.

If we don't evacuate our feces regularly, our bowels (or pipes) get plugged up. Where does the extra poop go? As previously mentioned, it becomes hardened, stagnant fecal matter that lingers inside our intestines. So if you are not having regular bowel movements, you are setting yourself up for sewage damage somewhere down the road. Having regular bowel movements and the right kind of stool is a way for you to monitor your status, ensuring you're not holding onto toxic matter that would otherwise be putrefying in your colon. This congestion also diminishes your capacity to absorb vital nutrients. Cleaning out your colon is a key place to start in regaining your health. Keep this exit route for wastes and toxins unencumbered.

Some people think that colonic irrigations are not natural and therefore should not be practiced. I guess we could say they are not natural, but neither is our modern-day way of eating. We eat things that our body has difficulty evacuating, therefore we need help to get things moving along. Emergency medical interventions are not natural either, but they can save people's lives. In the old days, doing enemas was an effective method to bring down a fever and also helped release a build-up of toxins that in turn permitted the body to heal itself from certain ailments, saving people's lives. This intervention can accomplish the same things today.

Alternative health professionals and health advocates have long been aware of the impressive health benefits of regularly cleaning out the colon. They are totally convinced that the health of the colon has a great impact on the health of the body. Dr. Norman Walker, author of *Colon Health: The Key to a Vibrant Life!* says:

*My study and intensive research on this subject convinces me more than ever that no treatment or healing procedure should **ever** be started without first giving the patient a series of colon irrigations in order to clean out the colon and remove the incipient source of infection. There is no ailment, sickness or disease that will not respond to treatment quicker and more effectively than it will after the administration of a series of colon irrigations.*[2]

Be assured, colonic irrigations can be a beneficial option in restoring your health.

THE KIDNEYS

One kidney is located just behind the liver on the right side of the body, the other just behind and slightly above the pancreas on the left side. Each one is about the size of a fist and each kidney contains about one million tiny filters made up of blood vessels. The main job of our urinary system is to remove waste products from the body, keeping toxins from building up in the bloodstream. The kidneys also help regulate the proper balance of minerals and electrolytes (salts), calcium and potassium, as well as maintain the correct levels of water in our body. They also produce hormones that control other bodily functions: regulating blood pressure, maintaining bone metabolism and producing red blood cells. Kidneys are very important organs.

After the blood has circulated through your body, it passes through your kidneys. The kidneys filter waste products, excess salt and water out of the blood and then pass these out as urine. If your bowels are not functioning well and toxins from your intestines are not being expelled sufficiently, it is only normal that your kidneys will have to work harder to compensate. Too many toxins can indeed damage the kidneys.

Most diseases of the kidneys attack the filtering units, called nephrons. Disease damages their ability to eliminate wastes and excess fluids, and then we get into a vicious circle of having too many toxic residues once again. Now another elimination organ is not able to eliminate properly. Usually, kidney disease starts slowly and silently and progresses over a number of years. This can lead to chronic kidney failure, which also happens gradually over a period of months to years.

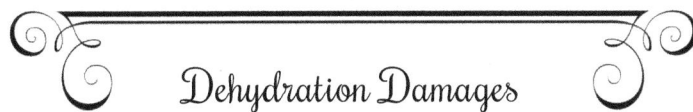

Dehydration Damages

Always drink plenty of clean, pure water. The formation of kidney stones in the kidney itself or in the urinary tract is most often caused by chronic dehydration.

Waste products that build up in the body cause imbalances in chemicals needed to keep the body functioning smoothly. It is a serious problem when the kidneys stop working. If the kidneys shut down for even a short time, a person can die of toxaemia or systemic toxicity. Dialysis may be urgently needed for a time. Thankfully, kidney failure can often be reversed if the underlying cause is treated on time.

THE LUNGS

Without sufficient oxygen, our body cannot properly utilise the food we eat and drink, even if the food is nourishing. Our body needs oxygen to burn, or metabolize, our food, just as in the example of our woodstove. We fan the flame of the fire to increase oxygen to make the fire burn better. The same goes for the metabolic process of our food.

Without a sufficient supply of oxygen, our bloodstream becomes saturated with poisonous carbon dioxide and other toxic wastes that keep accumulating as blood circulates throughout our whole body. These toxins are then brought back to the heart to be expelled through the lungs. If your breathing is shallow, if you lack exercise or fresh air, your cells are actually being suffocated instead of being rejuvenated with sufficient oxygen.

Subsequently, the blood loaded with an overabundant amount of toxins also has difficulty transporting the necessary nourishment from food to our cells. So, like our woodstove whose ashes are never removed, our body lacks oxygen and the flame of the fire gets dimmer and dimmer. A lack of oxygen slows down all of our bodily functions.

MAINTAINING ADEQUATE OXYGEN INTAKE

Shallow breathing, along with the wrong diet, causes our detoxing organs to be overworked and underfed. The problem is that accumulated wastes do not simply disappear—they will accumulate somewhere in the body. Additionally, when our body has too many toxins, our vital organs underperform, and we begin to develop such symptoms as headaches, fatigue and low immunity.

Other factors, other than shallow breathing, diminish our capacity for adequate oxygen intake. Eating junk food, which is refined and void of oxygen, on a regular basis forces the body to use up more of its oxygen reserves than usual to metabolize the preservatives, additives and what few nutrients may actually be in the food. Again as a reminder, the woodstove needs oxygen to burn the wood. We also need oxygen to digest, and metabolise, our food. Eating refined foods is not a good return on our investment – or rather for our ingestion. Refined sugar, white flour, alcohol, caffeinated beverages and soft drinks also rob oxygen from the body.

The body has to divert needed oxygen from primary metabolic functions – such as heartbeat, blood flow, brain function and immune response – just to oxidize and metabolize these foods.[3] Dense foods, such as fats and proteins, are also low in oxygen. Complex carbohydrates like raw fruits and raw vegetables, on the other hand, are very high in oxygen.

It's important to understand that a sedentary lifestyle can inhibit the removal of toxic wastes from your body, making you also prone to future illness. When you exercise, a generous flow of oxygen gets pumped into your body. Every cell becomes alive and invigorated, releasing even more energy for the exercise. That's why it's important to do your daily exercise routine no matter how tired you feel. You will always be thankful that you did because you will feel so much more energized afterwards. The increased supply of oxygen is also utilised by your body to help it detox even more. Oxygen is vital to detoxing, so you need to utilise your lungs to help detoxify your body. Deep breathing exercises and aerobic exercises are a must for a healthy body.

THE SKIN

The skin is actually the most expansive organ of our body. It protects the underlying muscles, bones, ligaments and internal organs. The skin is the membrane that separates our body from the exterior world. It prevents harmful bacteria from entering our body. Skin also functions as insulation, helps control temperature regulation and sensation, and is used in the production of our much-needed vitamin D.

Our skin is porous; it breathes. Toxic substances can penetrate our body via the skin. Chemically perfumed creams, as well as other harmful substances, can pass through our skin barrier through our pores, adding to our body's toxic load. Most people are not aware of this. As indicated in chapter 2, becoming aware and informed and then taking action to protect ourselves from undue exposure to chemical products is a huge step towards obtaining good health.

Yes, we absorb many harmful chemical substances through our skin, but the inverse is equally true: we also expel toxins through our skin. Waste is passed through the skin in the form of perspiration. Sweating is a very important part of detoxing. Because the skin is a very large organ, large amounts of toxins can flow out of our many pores. It's extremely important to use this detoxing vehicle, our skin, to sweat several times a week to flush out as many toxins as possible, thus relieving the workload on our other detoxing organs.

THE LIVER

The liver is on the upper right side of the abdomen, decreasing in size as it stretches across almost the entire width of the body. It's the largest internal organ of the body and a very important detoxifier.

Although the liver does not physically expel toxins from the inside of the body to the outside as the other four detoxifying organs do, it is a powerful inner detoxification organ. In fact, the liver is the dumping ground for all the toxins and chemicals that enter the body. It has the enormous job of deconstructing all of these substances, whether they enter from the outside through ingestion, respiration or through our skin, or whether they come from inside through the metabolizing process.

The liver is a highly complex organ. According to the Canadian Liver Foundation, it's responsible for more than 500 different functions, including the production of proteins and hormones, managing blood sugar, warding off infection and aiding with blood-clotting mechanisms.[4] It's also responsible for the converting of pharmaceutical drugs, or any other drug, into safer, broken down elements in order to complete the metabolism process.

Following the absorption of vitamins, minerals and all kinds of food additives including flavour enhancers, food coloring, preservatives, artificial sweeteners, chemicals used in agriculture and all other food molecules up through the small intestine, these substances immediately go to the liver for deconstruction, transformation or detoxing. The liver is responsible for diffusing, deconstructing and converting all toxins into substances that can be safely removed from the body. It also has to deal with by-products from our digestion. For example, ammonia is released with the digestion of protein. The liver converts this into a less toxic chemical compound called *urea*, which is then eliminated through the urine.

In general, wastes that the liver encounters are broken down or converted and are either carried out by bile into the small intestine or carried by the blood to be expelled by the kidneys or the lungs. Surplus toxic residue will be stored in fat cells. If there are too many toxic wastes for the liver to manage at one time, they recirculate into the blood and can damage other organs.

HELPING THE LIVER

When you are sick or fighting a degenerative disease, it's crucial to cut back on all chemical or toxic exposure. This includes cutting back on all processed foods, including processed meat. It's also a good idea to cut back on all meat and dairy products. Dairy products are very mucous forming and clog up our system. Meat protein has to be broken down by the liver into smaller amino acids so they can be used by the body. Therefore plant proteins are best, as they have already been broken down into the amino acids that are essential for assimilation. To give your liver less work to do, so that it can be more available to attend to the problem at hand, eat light foods, such as raw and steamed vegetables, along with soaked or sprouted nuts and seeds. Bitter plants, such as dandelion greens, watercress and arugula are also an excellent stimulus for the liver.

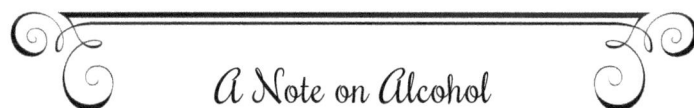
A Note on Alcohol

Alcohol that is not detoxified properly by the liver, because of liver overload, can cause serious injury and destroy liver cells. This is called cirrhosis of the liver. This means that the normally healthy liver cells have been damaged and replaced by scar tissue. This reduces the number of healthy cells remaining to perform their many important functions. A cirrhosis-damaged liver can cause disruption of many body functions and cause waste products to build up in the blood and tissues. Non-alcoholic fatty liver disease associated with obesity and diabetes can also cause liver cirrhosis.[5]

When there is an overabundance of toxic debris in the body and when the lungs don't receive enough oxygen, or if the bowels are congested and the kidneys are taxed or not working up to par, these toxins will keep flowing through the blood. Our incredibly resourceful body will urgently try to find other ways of getting rid of them. The liver will play a big part in this process. In particular, it might instruct the body to produce or hold on to fat in order to have a place to store the toxins. It can also utilise cholesterol molecules to capture and isolate these toxins and bacteria. These agglomerated cholesterol molecules mixed in with toxins and debris eventually develop into liver stones. A liver can contain thousands of these cholesterol-based stones. These stones, or rather globs, are not very dense, and so are not often picked up by X-ray machines. However, these small globs of bacteria-laden cholesterol block the functioning of the liver as well as the gall bladder and can lead to many health problems, such as: poor digestion, hormone imbalances, weight gain, fatigue, skin problems and chemical sensitivities.

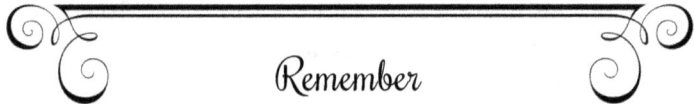

Remember

The liver is a manufacturing plant, a processing plant, a detoxification plant and much more. The activity in the liver is sometimes critically diminished by these cholesterol globules and can contribute to a diseased state.

We can do great harm to our liver by living an unhealthy lifestyle. However, our amazing liver is very resilient and can often be restored simply by stopping the inflow of destructive substances, increasing good, healthy foods and by going through a liver detox. In my opinion, we all need to do a deep liver cleanse once in our lives, at the very minimum. You must prepare your body for this by going on a detoxing diet, all the while taking therapeutic herbs to support your colon and your liver before doing the actual flush. There are several important factors to take into consideration as to the time you do this, so again, please get support from a qualified person.

The liver never stops working. It is one great detoxifying organ. Make sure it remains healthy so that it can do all of its complex jobs, including neutralizing wastes and deactivating toxins to ensure good health.

Please do not do a liver cleanse on your own. If your body is not prepared properly and your systemic evacuation routes are not open, you can put yourself in a worse condition and sometimes a dangerous mess. See a health professional, a naturopath or other alternative health care practitioner to assist you.

THE LYMPHATIC SYSTEM

The lymphatic system is a network of canals or vessels specially designed to deal with cellular debris, viruses and bacteria. It acts like an internal waste treatment system. It's armed with lymphocytes, which are white blood cells that make up the main part of the immune system. Lymph capillaries join together and become larger lymph vessels, which eventually dump back into the blood vessels in the large veins of the neck. In this way, the lymphatic system is part of the circulatory system, also known as the cardiovascular system.

The blood in the cardiovascular system is pushed through the body by a pump called the heart. In contrast, the lymphatic liquid (lymph), does not have a pump to push it through the lymph vessels. The only way the lymph can move is by the contraction of our muscles. This is why it is so important to get up, move around and exercise!

All cells are surrounded by fluid called interstitial fluid. This is where, in addition to blood capillaries, we find the lymph capillaries. Blood capillaries are very permeable and permit the nutrients, as well as toxins, present in the blood to seep into this interstitial fluid. The cells are then able to absorb these nutrients and begin whatever function or task each particular cell is designed to do. After these cells, or tiny manufacturing plants, have finished their work, they need to expel the residue (or ashes; woodstove, remember?) that the metabolizing process has produced. This residue and other toxins are then evacuated into the surrounding interstitial fluid.

The lymph's main job is to absorb this residue and debris found in the interstitial fluid. Some of these debris will be reabsorbed by the blood capillaries and returned to the heart to then be expelled by the lungs or kidneys. For the most part, however, debris is picked up by the lymph capillaries.

The lymph, like the liver, does not eliminate toxins from the inside to the outside of the body like the other detoxifying organs – the bowels, kidneys, lungs and skin. However, it is an important inner detoxifying system that plays a vital role in combatting disease. This is something that you should understand if you want to help your body to detoxify and be healthy.

THE LYMPH NODES

As the lymph gets pushed further and further along the lymph vessels, it will have passed through many filtering stations called lymph nodes. A lymph node is an oval-shaped organ that contains an even higher concentration of lymphocytes than in the lymphatic vessels. It is in these filtering stations that debris, bacteria and other pathogens are broken down and deactivated.

We have thousands of lymph nodes spread throughout our whole body, all interconnected to our lymph vessels. Many lymph nodes are grouped into clusters under the arms, and in the groin, neck and abdomen. It is in the lymph nodes that the battle against disease and infections takes place. These lymph nodes can be likened to small munitions factories. The more pathogens, the more the activity in the factory. They therefore become enlarged and inflamed when facing the overgrowth of pathogens from minor infections to serious diseases like cancer.

A HEALTHY LYMPH IS VITAL

The efficient working of our lymph system is critical in helping to eliminate disease. Firstly, we know that the lymph doesn't move if our body is inactive. It's the moving of our muscles that squeezes the lymph farther and farther up the network of lymph vessels through to the lymph nodes, our highly efficient filtering stations. If our body can't get the debris surrounding our cells into the lymph capillaries and up to the lymph nodes to deactivate and destroy pathogens, there will be a proliferation of bacteria, viruses and other debris. Our delicate cells will be bathing in toxins, no longer able to do their job adequately. That's when disease can silently begin to set in.

Having a daily exercise program is thus a proactive form of insurance for the prevention of disease. Exercise is important even when we are sick, even though it's the last thing we feel like doing. Of course, we must adjust the intensity to meet our particular health situation.

Healthy lymph has a liquid consistency; however, when we are unhealthy and disease ridden, our lymph has a thick, sticky consistency, which makes it even more difficult to move along through the various lymph nodes to be treated by the white blood cells of our immune system. Our unhealthy, high-sugar, highly refined carbohydrate, highly processed meat and dairy diet plugs up our lymph. These types of foods create thick, sticky lymph. The consumption of fruits and vegetables, especially raw, has the opposite effect on our lymph. Drinking sufficient amounts of pure water with the addition of half a lemon or lime squeezed in also helps break up the congestion and helps dilute the lymph so that it can circulate more efficiently. It is important to understand that a congested body leads to a diseased body.

OTHER WAYS THE BODY DEALS WITH EXCESS TOXINS

Our eliminating organs are not working sufficiently when we become constipated or when we don't have regular bowel movements, and when our kidneys are not able to eliminate residue as they should. Detoxification also does not occur properly when we aren't active physically, not sweating regularly and not breathing in abundant amounts of oxygen. If, added to all that, our liver is congested and rundown, and if we have thick, sticky, debris-laden, stagnant lymph, we will have a huge backup of harmful substances that are not being eliminated from our bodies. We then reach a point of saturation. When in this state, we are like a ticking time bomb. Debilitating disease is just around the corner.

However, our incredibly resilient body, ingeniously designed for survival, will begin to find other creative ways to try and hide these excess toxins and get them out of circulation.

We have already briefly talked about a resourceful place the body stores toxins: the fat cells. Ever wonder why some people have a hard time losing weight? Even if they hardly eat anything, that weight just won't come off. It's not always because that person eats too much; it could rather be due to the kind of foods he or she eats. If the food this person is eating is acidic or contains a lot of toxic chemical products, even if he or she eats little, weight loss can become very difficult. Disregarding the hormonal disruption that comes from eating a diet high in processed carbohydrates and high in acidic foods, which in itself causes stubborn weight loss challenges, there also may simply be too many acidic toxins stored in the fat. The body will not let go of them for fear of too many toxins being released into the blood stream, entering tissues and potentially destroying organs. Remember, our body will do everything to survive; even if it means keeping us fat.

Another place our body stores toxins is in the joints. Have you ever had stiff joints? It's not always because of the wear and tear of old age; it could very well be due to acidity and toxins. These toxins can accumulate over the years; so the older we get, the more toxic accumulation and acidity, the more damage it can cause, the more it hurts. With time this condition can end up in arthritis. The body uses the calcium from the bones to neutralize these acidic toxins. This in turn forms tiny calcium crystals that damage our joints and also causes inflammation. Also know that extreme, repetitive exercise or living with chronic stress can likewise contribute to the premature deterioration of our cartilage especially in combination with a highly acidic diet.

> YOUR BODY STORES HARMFUL TOXINS IN FAT CELLS AND JOINTS

Cysts, colds, mucous and other small signs like dandruff, excessive amounts of wax in our ears, smelly feet – can all be signs of the body trying to expel extra toxins or debris. These are some of the red warning lights on our body's dashboard that are beginning to flicker.

THE CONSEQUENCES OF OVERACIDIFICATION

Our amazing body will not only try to excrete or hide overabundant, harmful substances, but will even try to neutralize these toxins. Toxins are acidic. Foods such as red meat and dairy, wheat, chips, soda pop, coffee and alcohol, are also acidic. Minerals such as calcium, potassium and magnesium – which are mainly found in vegetables – are alkaline. These minerals are particularly effective in neutralizing the acidity in our bodies. If we don't have enough of these minerals from our diet to do this job, the body leaches calcium out of the bones and even the teeth, or it leaches magnesium from the muscles and uses that to neutralise the acidity. This can lead to deficiencies in the body, creating many varied symptoms. One well-known symptom is called osteoporosis.

The blood always keeps itself in balance; the technical term is called *homeostasis*. If it gets too acidic or out of balance, the body will not be able to remain alive, so it does everything it can to maintain the required pH level. Even if it means leaching calcium from the bones.

Our blood is ideally maintained at a pH of 7.365. The blood must maintain or remain very close to this pH level or we are at risk of death, but this is not true of our tissues. Our tissues can become very acidic. The body pulls out minerals from our organs and tissues to maintain the critical blood pH level of 7.365. When the body performs this function to ensure survival, it leaves our organs and tissues in an acidic state.[6] However, our body cannot undergo long periods of time with this acid-base imbalance without our organs and tissues weakening and eventually succumbing to disease. In his book *The pH Miracle*, Dr. Robert Young wrote the following:

> *The pH level of our internal fluids affects every cell in our body. The entire metabolic process depends on an alkaline environment. Chronic over-acidity corrodes body tissue and if left unchecked will interrupt all cellular activities and functions, from the beating of your heart to the neural firing of your brain. In other words, over acidity interferes with life itself. It is at the root of all sickness and disease.*[7]

Excess acidity in the body, with the exception of the stomach, is extremely harmful. We don't feel the acidity in our organs and tissues *per se*, so we don't worry too much about it. Over time, however, as our organs become more and more acidic they become more and more nutrient deficient and no longer able to function at optimum levels.

TREATING OVERACIDIFICATION

Now you know that to prevent degenerative diseases, the cells and tissues of your body must be in an alkaline state. So how do you measure the pH level of your tissues and organs? You can measure your own saliva and urine pH with Litmus™ paper strips. Saliva is too fluctuant and so not a very reliable way to indicate true tissue acidity. Using Litmus® paper strips to test urine samples is more reliable, though not always 100% accurate. Another way of deducing if your organs are in an acidic state is to look at what you eat and to observe your level of stress. If you eat a lot of processed foods, including fast foods, drink a lot of coffee and soft drinks, eat refined carbohydrates, a lot of sweets, too much meat and don't eat an adequate amount of vegetables – especially dark leafy green vegetables which are full of alkaline minerals–on a regular basis, your tissues and organs are most certainly in an acidic state. It's only a question of time before you will fall prey to some kind of dis-ease or even degenerative disease.

Acidity in your body irritates your organs and tissues, which in turn causes inflammation. You want to do all you can to reverse your cellular acidity problem before it causes multiple long-term damage. You can do this through eating a more alkaline diet, exercising regularly and reducing stress. Please, especially do not neglect eating your alkalinizing greens!

A WORD ON ACID REFLUX

Acid reflux is simply our body emitting a warning sign: something's not going right. There are several different causes of acid reflux. One is physical pressure being put on the lower oesophageal valve, allowing acid from the stomach to leak out, either from being overweight or from pregnancy. Quite surprisingly, acid reflux is often due to our stomach not producing enough hydrochloric acid.

Overeating may also cause acid reflux as improperly treated and digested food is not ready to leave the stomach to continue on towards the small intestine. The over consumption of refined carbohydrates (refined starches), as well as their improper digestion can cause excess fermentation which then creates a pressure in the digestive tract, causing acid reflux as well as reducing our hydrochloric acid levels. Chronic stress may likewise contribute to your less-than optimal stomach acid levels.

Many people turn to antacids in order to remove the acidity that is burning their esophagus or to relieve other uncomfortable symptoms related to heart burn. Although one may receive immediate relief of the effects of acidity, in the long term, antacids in any form makes the situation worse. They lower the acidity that is needed to digest our food properly.

Long term usage of antacids chronically lowers our stomach acid levels which causes bacterial overgrowth. This may lead to candida and leaky gut syndrome. Certain bacterial overgrowth, in particular *H. pylori* (Helicobacter pylori), may even cause stomach ulcers that may then lead to cancer. Thus, long term usage of antacids are not recommended for the treatment of acid reflux.

Eating alkaline vegetables along with your consumption of meat or starchy carbohydrates can reduce acid reflux. The digestion of vegetables does not deplete our hydrochloric acid like proteins and carbs do. Ostensibly, with an increased consumption of vegetables we will eat less meats and carbs, thereby requiring less hydrochloric acid.

Drinking a bit of apple cider vinegar in a small amount of water before meals helps with digestion. Beets are also great for stimulating the production of hydrochloric acid levels, as are salt, iodine and zinc. Periodical supplementation with hydrochloric acid drops or tablets helps to increase low stomach acid.

CYSTS

Cysts and tumors can be found on the ovaries, kidneys or in virtually any part of your body. Although there are many different kinds of cysts, doctors consider many to be idiopathic, which means they generally form for unknown reasons. Skin cysts that can be described as non-cancerous are enclosed parcels of tissue filled with fluid, pus or other bodily material.[8] The many cysts that are filled with a mixture of fats, captured bacteria and toxins is the way the body captures, isolates and removes unneeded or damaging substances from circulation. I believe this is simply a creative strategy of the body for putting in place mechanisms to deal with the overload of toxic matter or residue coming from the environment and from an unhealthy lifestyle. These cysts may appear from exposure to environmental chemicals, processed foods and other foreign elements as well as to chronic stress and toxic emotions. All of this, when accompanied with a sedentary lifestyle, congests our lymph and undermines the proper functioning and detoxifying of our body.

Always include some kind of raw vegetable at each of your meals to ensure a sufficient supply of minerals. This also serves to counteract the acidity coming from the consumption of processed foods, refined carbohydrates or an excessive amount of protein that you may presently find difficult eliminating from your diet. Raw veggies also contribute to increased oxygen in the body. This practice also supplies the body with much needed enzymes as well as fibre that helps clean the colon and remove toxins

SUMMARY

- **Given the proper environment, the body is well equipped to heal quickly and naturally on its own.** When functioning properly and given the right nutritional support as well as being in a relaxed mental and emotional state, the four eliminating organs (colon, kidneys, lungs and skin) as well as the liver and the lymph system together, are able to purge our body of many of the toxins we've been exposed to.

- **Our bodies pay the price of our bad choices**. We flush our system of impurities through our four eliminating organs as well as our liver and our lymph. However, if we are not able to do so adequately due to congestion in the body, and when there's an overabundance of these harmful substances flowing in, our body begins to manifest the consequences. With time, if we go on ignoring these warning signs, they will become louder and louder and more and more intense until we find ourselves well on the road to contracting all kinds of degenerative diseases.

- **It is crucial that our body maintains its capacity to detox regularly**. Committing to a healthier lifestyle, which includes regular physical activity as well as drinking plenty of water, is crucial to supporting our body's natural detoxification systems.

As we will see in the next chapter, learning to recognize when our body is beginning to malfunction and applying proper intervention can stop the progression of disease.

4

CHAPTER FOUR

Dashboard lights and degenerative diseases

So far we've elaborated on nutritional deficiency, the overload of toxins in our food and in our environment, stress as well as how the body eliminates toxins. We now know that we are well equipped to remove toxins from our body.

However, when we overload our system with processed food, junk food and other chemical and toxic substances, the body is unable to effectively remove these impurities. When things get backed up, we get sick. Most of us are oblivious to initial warning signs like: skin problems, lethargy, brain fog, joint problems or weight-gain, etc. Over time, if we continue to let these things go unchecked, we may ultimately end up with a debilitating, degenerative disease, such as diabetes, heart disease or cancer. In this chapter we will observe what happens when we ignore these initial warning signs and what the consequences are of being negligent regarding the health of our body and that of our future generations.

When we consider and try to understand these initial signs and when we start to take responsibility for our health, giving our body what it needs to be healthy and doing what is necessary to help it detoxify, amazing things can happen. Let's dive in so that we can better understand how we can make these changes. We have more control over our health than we think.

WARNING SIGNS ON YOUR DASHBOARD

All cars are equipped with a dashboard. A dashboard provides warning signs and red lights to let you know that there is some kind of problem. Imagine you are headed on a long journey. You jump into your car and, after a short time, begin to have car problems. I don't think many of you would continue to drive if a red light was to suddenly pop up indicating engine problems, or a bell would begin to ring reminding you that you are nearing the end of your fuel. It wouldn't make too much sense to continue. Even if you pushed and kept on going as though nothing were wrong, you would definitely not reach your destination.

This is what happens with your body. Your body is your vehicle. Amazingly, your body is also equipped with a dashboard indicating all kinds of dis-ease: headaches, joint stiffness, sharp or gnawing pain, shortness of breath, fatigue, weight gain, constipation, acne, heartburn, expanding waist line and so on. The problem is that many of us have not really learned to see, listen to or heed these warning signs. Rather, we have learned to deny, disregard, misinterpret, misdiagnose or simply accept them; consequently, we do not take proper action.

If these signs are aggravating enough and possibly because we are looking for a quick fix, we let ourselves be convinced by keen advertisements that some kind of magic pill or other "Band-Aid" treatment will get rid of this warning light or another. Sometimes we get relief, but it's often only temporary. Taking a pill or medication to treat a symptom without also looking for and dealing with the initial cause of the problem, is equivalent to putting masking tape on the red warning icon on your dashboard, or even ripping out the wiring that connects the problem to the ringing bell. It may mask the pain or the symptom, but it doesn't deal with the root issue. Actions like these may make us feel as though we are heading in the right direction. After all, the pain has been alleviated. But then, we forget about addressing what caused the problem in the first place. Depending on our circumstances and situation, over time there may be another red light, or another bell ringing.

We continue, sometimes for years, with the same procedure, masking or disconnecting the link to our problem until finally we succumb to some debilitating disease. When sickness hits, we pray with all our might for a miracle to happen, never realizing that many times it has been the cumulative, repetitive, negative lifestyle choices and the stressful or harmful situations that we have been exposed to that have led us to where we are today.

Be reassured, miracles do happen. I believe in prayer and I believe in miracles. However, there are no guarantees for receiving a miraculous healing. On the other hand, the rectification of our negative lifestyle habits can give us a huge advantage to help us gain our health back. Why not do both: make healthy lifestyle changes and pray? I believe that we can experience a miracle every single time we eat food for which our body was created. Our miraculous body goes to work using nature's whole, live foods to in turn give us sustained health, vitality and energy.

> YOU MAY FEEL LIKE YOU ARE HEADED IN THE RIGHT DIRECTION WHILE MOVING RAPIDLY TOWARD A DEAD END

Our body is resilient and can bounce back quickly. This happens when we stop the intake of pernicious foods and don't expose ourselves to other harmful substances, including our negative emotions. Instead, we provide beneficial, wholesome foods and walk with a joyful spring in our step.

So many people are being afflicted and dying of such atrocious diseases, young people included. Some people believe that sickness and disease is God's will. Is this really true? I don't think so. God is good. How can a loving God possibly be the instigator of something so destructive? We need to face the fact that, in most cases, it's possible that our negative lifestyle choices and our unconscious negative beliefs are the greatest contributors to our ill health.

A Note on Public Health

Sometimes we look at the masses eating sub-optimal foods and living sedentary lifestyles, and because they don't appear to be sick, we think that we also can make these same choices without incurring any major negative consequences. However, just take a

> *couple of minutes to really think about these same people. Are you sure they are healthy? Actually, do you know of anyone without a health problem? Or anyone without some ache or pain? The reality is that our society, for the most part, is not healthy because it does not eat well enough. Most people have health challenges. Some may not be aware of them simply because the symptoms haven't fully manifested themselves yet.*

In today's modern society, chronic degenerative diseases increase with age. How many people do you know over the age of 65 who don't have at least one chronic illness; asthma, emphysema or rheumatoid arthritis; or are on some type of medication whether it be for high blood pressure, diabetes, cholesterol or the like? Today, I don't think anyone would think that it's abnormal to die of a disease. In fact, in 2004, according to "The Surgeon General's Report on Nutrition and Health", 89% of Americans died from a degenerative disease![1] Degenerative disease increases with age because we have had many more years of accumulated waste and chemical toxins contaminating and burdening our bodies; years of either seemingly innocuous or perhaps more obviously poor eating habits, chronic stress and sedentary lifestyles. Growing old is natural and normal, but growing old and being stricken with degenerative diseases is not. It doesn't have to be this way. It should be normal to just die of old age.

We personally have a big part to play in our having good health through making consistent, disciplined, healthy choices every day throughout our entire life. Taking responsibility for our own health empowers us. How do we do this? Being open and curious about how our body works and what it needs to be healthy and then taking steps to get informed, is a good place to start. You are doing just that as you read this book–congratulations! Don't stop here, keep learning and then apply what you learn.

We can also take responsibility by becoming aware when our body is giving us signs and signals that something is going wrong. We then can begin to make small, incremental adjustments to our diet and lifestyle accordingly. In Part 2 of this book we will be going over some basic principles and steps to help us move towards good health. But for now, let's hold our course in order to fully understand what contributes to our being sick so that we can be better equipped and motivated to make those necessary changes. Knowledge empowers!

EPIGENETICS

Some may think that their sickness is genetic and therefore they are simply victims condemned to contracting the same disease or illness as their parents or grandparents. However, there is a new emerging science called *epigenetics* that is in the process of discovering and confirming that our diseases may not be genetically passed down in the way we have previously believed.

It seems that certain characteristics of our genes can be activated or deactivated depending on different factors coming from the environment. According to an article from the *Mayo Clinic Health Letter* regarding epigenetics, healthy diets combined with a balanced lifestyle as well as a positive attitude, ensures the activation of the healthy part of our genetic code.[2] The flip side of this is that harmful environmental factors such as chemical toxins, bad diet and sedentary lifestyle habits along with negative thought patterns such as anxiety and stress, may determine the activation of the part of our gene which initiates disease. Consequently, even if we have been genetically pre-disposed to certain diseases, we may no longer be victims to these diseases if we take preventive measures to give to our cells (our genes are contained in the DNA of our cells) what they need to be healthy.

We can now confirm that we are not necessarily the victim of "bad genes" being passed down, but perhaps it's the modelling of an unhealthy lifestyle that has been passed down to us. Regardless, the science of epigenetics helps us affirm that having a balanced, healthy lifestyle does help protect our health, either by activating the healthy genetic program of our genes or by deactivating the negative genetic program that is responsible for manifesting disease. Being proactive with our diet and lifestyle can push back disease. There is hope we can change things around.

WHAT ARE DEGENERATIVE DISEASES?

According to the *Mosby's Medical Dictionary*, the definition of degenerative disease is: "Any disease in which deterioration of structure or function of tissue occurs." Kinds of degenerative diseases include arteriosclerosis, cancer and osteoarthritis.[3] Degenerative diseases are non-infectious and are not caused by viruses. Basically, it's the body breaking down because of nutrient deficiencies and toxic overload causing damage to our cells and tissues through oxidation and inflammation.

MAIN DEGENERATIVE DISEASES IN OUR SOCIETY TODAY

Degenerative diseases can be divided into several major groups: cardiovascular diseases, neoplastic diseases, diseases of the nervous system and degenerative bone and joint diseases. Following are a few examples of each.

CARDIOVASCULAR DISEASES

- Hypertension or high blood pressure
- Heart disease, including coronary disease (narrowing of the arteries) and heart attacks
- Cerebrovascular accidents (CVAs or strokes)

NEOPLASTIC DISEASES

- Benign tumours
- Cancers

DISEASES OF THE NERVOUS SYSTEM

- Alzheimer's disease
- Parkinson's disease

DEGENERATIVE BONE AND JOINT DISEASES

- Osteoporosis
- Rheumatoid arthritis

According to the 2015 annual worldwide figures from the World Health Organization (WHO), the following are some of the leading causes of premature death:[4]

- Ischaemic heart disease (8.76 million)
- Cancer (8.8 million)[5]
- Stroke (6.24 million)
- Respiratory infections (3.19 million)
- Diabetes (1.59 million)

The Centers for Disease Control and Prevention (CDC) published a report showing that diabetes is on the rise, almost tripling between 1990 and 2010. Type 2 diabetes accounts for 95% of diagnosed diabetes in adults, while 5% have type 1. The same report stated that if this trend continues, one in three U.S. adults could find themselves with type 2 diabetes by the year 2050.[6] The number of Canadians with type 2 diabetes is also on the rise, with 60,000 new cases added each year.[7] This does not include the many people who have diabetes but are not aware of their condition.

This is disturbing because there are crippling consequences to having long-term diabetes. Many people who have diabetes also have heart disease. The American Heart Association stated that: "At least 68% of people age 65 or older with diabetes die from heart disease and 16% die of stroke."[8] Diabetes can also lead to amputation, blindness and kidney failure.

As we can see, degenerative diseases are ever-present in our society today, destroying the lives of our friends and family. This is alarming and not normal. However, we can use this wakeup call to prompt us to become proactive in managing our health.

OBESITY

We have been led astray by the food industry and governmental agencies into consuming large quantities of unnatural and unhealthy products. Quite a few years back the *Food Guide Pyramid* had us eating 6 to 11 servings of food in the bread, cereal, rice and pasta group.[9] Most of the foods in this food group were refined grains that contribute to obesity and diabetes. There was no discrimination made between eating white rice and brown rice, and no emphasis made on eating alternatives to processed white flour products, such as whole grains, quinoa, amaranth or buckwheat. We need carbohydrates, but not from processed grain products. Anyone trying to follow the *Food Guide* back then may have gotten into the habit of eating a lot of unhealthy, high-glycemic foods.

Processed foods are not real foods, and eating large quantities of them not only makes us put on weight but also makes us ill. This is happening wherever there is an over-consumption of refined carbohydrates and processed foods, and where people are not partaking in regular exercise. William Reymond in his book *Toxic* declares: "There is no state in the world where obesity is not on the increase." He also clearly demonstrates that we are now facing a global obesity epidemic.[10]

It is interesting to note that we are the only mammals confused about what we should eat. There is a connection here. Natural laws and principles that govern the health of our body and the past proven traditions of our grandparents and great-grandparents have been laid by the wayside. It's no longer normal to abide by these principles and traditions. Instead, we rely on contradicting science and government to provide us with information on how to eat healthily.

> WE ARE THE ONLY MAMMALS ON THE PLANET CONFUSED ABOUT WHAT WE SHOULD EAT

There is always new scientific research telling us that we should eat a certain kind of food – but a few years later we are informed that we should be eating the opposite. Years ago we were informed that we should not eat egg yolks because they were high in cholesterol and could lead to heart attacks. Eggs are a very nutritious whole food, especially if they come from pasture-fed chickens. Eating peanut butter with added hydrogenated oils provides a much greater chance of causing cholesterol or heart problems than eating eggs does. Such contradicting information has brought about a lot of confusion. We have lost our ability to inherently know what is good for us.

METABOLIC SYNDROME AND DIABETES

One of the perilous problems with being overweight is that it can lead to what is called metabolic syndrome, which in turn leads to diabetes. One of the visible risk factors to having metabolic syndrome is the accumulation of fat, specifically around the abdomen. This indicator may also be accompanied by raised blood glucose levels, high blood pressure, high blood levels of triglycerides, or low levels of high-density lipoprotein (HDL-"good" cholesterol). Having three or more of these factors often indicates a higher risk of cardiovascular disease as well as type 2 diabetes.

Metabolic syndrome, or the accumulation of fat around the abdomen, is so prevalent in our North American society; its negative effects leads to such serious consequences that some doctors now call it "fat that kills."[11] Generally this is caused by the overconsumption of sugar as well as processed refined carbohydrates like bread, pasta, pastries, etc., also known as high-glycemic foods, along with a sedentary lifestyle. Many people who have metabolic syndrome are actually unaware of their condition, as they may have become accustomed to the visible symptom – the accumulation of fat around the waist – that in most cases has developed slowly but steadily over time.

The consumption of high glycemic foods leads to high blood sugar, which, over the years, can eventually lead to diabetes. However it is during this time (the metabolic syndrome phase, also known as the pre-diabetic phase) that complications associated with diabetes perniciously begin to develop, such as nerve damage, retinal damage, early signs of kidney deterioration, as well as the beginning of damage to arteries.

If you think that you eat a healthy balanced diet, but your waist measurement has been increasing over time, then you need to stop and reconsider the food you are eating as well as increase your physical activity. The same applies if you have high blood sugar issues. These signs are acting as red warning lights on your dashboard – your body is sending you signals! If you don't do something different in regard to your diet and lifestyle now, you may well be on your way to contracting full-blown diabetes and even cardiovascular disease in the not-so-distant future.

The thing with diabetes is that this disease doesn't seem that harmful in the beginning stages. You can just take a pill or an injection of insulin, and because of these interventions you don't necessarily have to make any changes to your diet. This can lead you to believe that you can continue to eat like you always have. This is very misleading. Eating high glycemic carbohydrates causes blood sugar imbalance and this keeps you in a vicious circle, causing you to remain dependant on insulin medication in order to regulate the issue. In other words, not changing your diet is keeping you in a diabetic or pre-diabetic state. Because your blood sugar has now been regulated by medicine it gives you the impression that everything is ok. This is just an illusion, as it has not dealt with the root problem.

If you decide to face this disease and make those necessary dietary changes, I can guarantee you will not regret it. Diabetes in the long term is a terribly debilitating disease that you want to avoid at all costs. It does take courage and determination, but you can turn type 2 diabetes around. Of course it is easier to do so in the beginning stages of diabetes and even easier in the metabolic syndrome phase, but regardless it's never too late.

To see how six people reversed their diabetes, view the documentary video available online: *Simply Raw: Reversing Diabetes in 30 Days*.

You don't have to be overweight or have an expanding waistline to have metabolic syndrome or diabetes. It's much less common, but even skinny people can suffer from type 2 diabetes. Stress and inflammation play a big part in this.

To be healthy we need to be eating 6 to 11 – or more – servings of food from the whole carbohydrates food group: lettuce, celery, bell peppers, broccoli, kale, tomatoes, carrots, spinach, squash, peas, apples, etc. These are whole, natural foods that come straight from nature. The old 1992 food pyramid recommended only 3 to 5 servings from this vegetable group per day. So by following this *Food Guide*, we were guided into eating the wrong quantities of food as well as the wrong kinds of carbohydrates. These unbalanced portions have now become an ingrained way of eating in our present society.

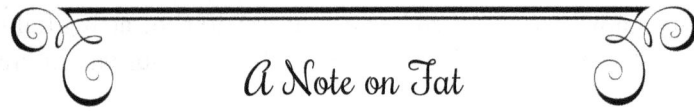

A Note on Fat

The emphasis on 0% fat is another conflicting and confusing subject. We are denaturing whole foods by taking out their natural fats. If we remove fats from something like natural yoghurt, for instance, something else must be added to retain the texture and taste. It's often cornstarch (a refined carbohydrate) or sugar, often both. We must realize that the "low fat" fad – the restriction of fats in our diet – is causing an increase in the consumption of high-glycemic foods which leads to weight gain and diabetes. Fat does not make you fat!

In fact, fat makes you healthy. Good fats are crucial for the proper functioning of our metabolism. Fat also helps insulin regulation. Some now say that our diets should be made up of 50% and up to 70% fat.[12] Some of the best sources include organic butter from raw milk, (unheated) virgin olive oil, coconut oil, raw nuts like pecans and macadamia nuts, free-range eggs, avocado, and wild Alaskan salmon.

Because we eat so many refined carbohydrates such as pasta, bread, crackers, cookies, cakes, donuts, etc., we are neither thriving nor healthy and we are slowly becoming more and more overweight. These foods fill us up and give us a feeling of satiation, but they also burden our bodies. One thing they do not do is nourish us adequately. As a result of nutrient-deficient diets, our immune system is slowly deteriorating.

> PROCESSED FOODS ARE NOT REAL FOODS

GLUTEN-FREE PRODUCTS

"Gluten-free" simply means that there is no gluten in any of the grains that are used to make bread for example. Some people suffer from a gluten allergy or intolerance. They are therefore turning to gluten-free flour products. However, these products are just as stripped of their nutrients as normal wheat products are. Additionally, gluten-free flour products may be just as acidic and may equally spike your blood sugar. Choosing a diet based on too many refined carbohydrates, whether gluten-free or not, causes health problems. Let's be creative and try new ways of eating.

CANCER

Cancer is also a form of disease heavily influenced by our diets and lifestyle choices, including our conscious and unconscious thoughts and emotions. Cancer cells want to live like any other cells do. They simply are cells that have adapted to live in an acidic, anaerobic environment. They cannot live in an alkaline environment but they proliferate in an acidic terrain.

Although most cells need oxygen to live, cancer cells have adapted to life with little oxygen. They compensate by developing many more glucose receptors; they live off of sugar. To keep cancer cells from growing and proliferating, cancer patients must radically change their diet to eliminate sugars, which includes refined carbohydrates. They also need to eliminate denatured processed foods, which are also very acidifying for the body. Cancer patients have lost their acid-base (or pH) equilibrium. They don't have the luxury of eating whatever they want. If they want to put all odds on their side, they need to use strategy and discipline. A big part of the strategy is to be able to reverse the acidic state of their bodies. They need to starve those cancer cells (no sugar, including all refined carbohydrates), rebuild the healthy cells and bring the alkalinity of the body back up. This can be done through diet.

Cancer patients especially must radically boost their raw vegetable intake. Juicing is a great way to increase nutritional intake and also greatly increases alkalinity. You will find a list of alkaline versus acidic foods in chapter 6 (Part 2 of this book). Another equally important part of this strategy is to be surrounded by a lot of love and support because they will need to address some of the unresolved emotional issues that are often times at the root of this disease.[13]

MY BROTHER'S STORY

To emphasize how important diet is to fighting cancer and disease, I'd like to share the story of my brother's fight with cancer.

My brother received a diagnosis of a slow-growing cancer called *medullary carcinoma* over 20 years ago. It's a rare type of thyroid cancer that cannot be treated by radiation or chemotherapy. Consequently, he had his cancerous thyroid gland removed. Over the years he had several other operations to remove the tumour, but it kept growing back. The doctors said that my brother could hope to live at most 7 to 15 years. They also warned him that this type of cancer would be accompanied by chronic diarrhoea. During this time my brother worked hard on trying to find the emotional root cause for this disease. He did a lot of deep personal work and was able to resolve a lot of emotional issues. He later began to work on changing his diet. He did some vegetable juicing on and off and tried to incorporate more raw foods, salads and other veggies along with some fresh fruit into his diet. Nonetheless, he also nourished his carbohydrate addiction: he loved his cup of coffee and cookies.

He undertook several detoxing treatments over the years. The growth of the cancer seemed to have been kept at bay. For many years the doctors were surprised that he did not have chronic diarrhoea. However, in the last few years of my brother's life, the tumour began growing bigger and bigger, and this time it started pushing on his oesophagus. Several times he experienced a bit of difficulty breathing.

The doctors said there was nothing they could do, only that if it got really bad, they could perform a tracheotomy. The operation involves placing a tube in the trachea or windpipe of the neck to permit airflow so the patient can breathe.

It must be a big challenge living with the threat of cancer taking your life for so many years. It had now been over 20 years since he was first diagnosed. I presume he had dropped his guard on his eating to heal and just wanted to live a normal life. I'm assuming it was at this time that he started having bouts of diarrhoea. He remembered that the doctors had said that this was the consequence of this type of cancer. So he just put up with it. He concentrated on helping people around him and totally focused on that.

NATURAL TREATMENTS

One summer when I came to visit my family, my brother was having 12 to 15 bouts of diarrhoea per day. He was an amazingly strong and resilient person. You would have never known that he had this problem for the past three years. I was worried for him and hoped to encourage him to take his health in hand and go on an alkalizing diet. Unfortunately, before I got there, his body had started to seriously decline. He had just moved from one city to another. This challenging relocation had caused him to go through an enormous amount of stress. He relied on lots of coffee drinking to help keep himself energized during this move. Because coffee is a diuretic, he came down with severe dehydration, causing the development of oedema (swelling) in his legs.

When I had arrived, he asked me to do anything I could to help him. I suggested that he get on a more alkaline diet to get rid of his oedema. I took him off all processed foods: no soft drinks, no Gatorade®, no bread, no processed wheat products, very little meat. I started giving him potassium soup, soup with lots and lots vegetables, especially green vegetables along with fresh vegetable juices and some therapeutic herbs to strengthen his organs.

I accompanied my brother to his various doctors' appointments. I asked the doctor how long it would take to get rid of his oedema. He told me that he would never get rid of it. I was surprised, as I knew that given the right elements, the body could heal itself and the oedema would disappear. It got worse before it got better. But it did get better. The oedema had gone past his knees and had almost reached his groin area. He was still walking and moving about, but with a lot of difficulty – that's a lot of extra weight on the legs.

I continued with the alkaline diet, a lot of raw and cooked vegetables, fresh vegetable juices and some fruit. In a few weeks, his oedema started to go down. Gradually, the retention of water in his legs decreased. It finally dropped back down to below his knees. One morning he woke up and the oedema had totally disappeared from his legs! He still had a bit of swelling in his feet, but his toes were nowhere swollen to the size they once were. Amazing. He was thrilled, and so was I. The doctor was baffled; he didn't know what to say.

One day, one of my brother's good friends came to see him. After they had spent a few hours visiting, when she was ready to leave, she gave him a hug and realized that his neck, which was so swollen just a few weeks before, had shrunk to about a third of what it was. This mass, which was so big that it was pushing on his oesophagus and beginning to impair his breathing, was now the size of an over-sized walnut. We were so amazed! I had put him on an alkaline diet to get rid of the oedema and, lo and behold, his cancer started to shrink. Every day from then on we noticed slower, but continual, diminishing of the tumour.

There was one more incredible development. About two weeks after I had started him on a healthy, natural diet, he told me: "Oh, by the way, my diarrhoea has been cut down from over 12 to 6 per day." That's over half of what it was. And another week later, it had decreased to 3 episodes, and he even started to pass a couple of loosely formed stools.

I was not trying to shrink his cancerous tumour or even trying to get rid of his diarrhoea. I was just trying to get the oedema in his legs down so that we could get him on the plane and continue his detoxifying program at my home. You see, when you give good, healthy nutrients to your body, it doesn't just use it to heal the parts of the body that you have in mind – it goes to work to heal the whole body. Our bodies are truly incredible.

A SAD ENDING

Unfortunately, several weeks later, my brother was hospitalized, as he no longer had muscle energy to carry himself around or even to sit himself up. We were not equipped to help him at home. His potassium levels were critically low. The doctors had him on potassium intravenously as well as orally. We continued to bring him green smoothies, homemade soups and real food for every meal; it was a huge effort for all of us. I am so proud of my family and how we all pulled together, each doing his or her part to do whatever we could for him. But even with all the work everyone put in, his body had deteriorated and could not hold on to the potassium. Lack of potassium affects muscle tonicity. He was having a hard time eating and drinking because the swallowing process also involves muscle tonicity.

Our whole family and his close friends can all have the sense that we did all that we could to help him. I know that he felt our love. One nurse commented that in all of her 25 years of nursing, she had never felt so much love walking into a hospital room as she did into his.

After three days of not eating or drinking, my dear brother quietly and peacefully passed away knowing that he was deeply loved. He touched many people's lives, and that love was coming back around, especially in the last months of his life. Unfortunately, his chronic diarrhoea, over time, had not allowed his intestines to absorb the nutrients his body needed to restore itself; they simply passed down his intestines too quickly. This impeded the absorption of vital nutrients. By the time he changed to a healthier diet his organs were already critically deteriorated and were not able to handle the release of the toxins from the oedema and from the disappearing tumour.

LESSONS LEARNED

The first lesson of this story is that the body cannot be separated into compartments. When we give good food to one part of the body, the nutrients automatically go to all the other parts. This is also true when taking prescription drugs or other medications. There are always negative side effects when taking medications. Even though they target specific parts of the body, they not only act upon the part of the body that is being treated; medication will also have some kind of impact on the rest of the body.

In naturopathy, we don't look at the body as having separate parts. We don't treat diseases as such, but rather we seek to treat root causes. We can then give the body what it needs. It is astonishing to see how so often it will heal itself. I am slightly oversimplifying, but it is to emphasize the importance of the fact that it is not so complicated after all. We don't have to understand everything in order to get results. Feed your body the nutrients it needs and surprisingly, it can recover by itself.

The second lesson to this story is don't wait till the last minute to start making changes in order to heal. If my brother had taken this radical stand to detoxify and heal his body three years earlier, before his chronic diarrhoea set in, his organs would have no doubt been in better condition to handle the detox. Perhaps he would still be here today helping people out, as he so loved to do.

MY BROTHER'S LEGACY

One thing I do want to say is that even if, in my eyes, my brother died prematurely, he passed away having first discovered his life purpose. Yes, he had stepped into his mission. After many years of struggling with his own issues, he learned from them, grew because of them and then went on to help others. It was from his own personal experience that he had developed into the extraordinary life coach that he was. He had an incredible way of making people feel validated, accepted and loved. With that foundation he was able to help people get through major roadblocks in their own personal lives. He did an incredible job of listening to, helping, loving and empowering others.

Six months before his passing, he told me that he knew what his mission on this earth was and that he was laser focused on that and did not want to waste one minute. He wanted to touch all the lives that he could before he left this world. He did. He left his mark with everyone that he came in contact with even until his last days. He was always so kind and considerate and had an incredible capacity for making people feel extra-special. He affirmed them and loved them unconditionally. We received so many moving and loving words from his clients. He was much loved because he was able to love much. We dearly miss him. It's unfortunate, but because of not understanding how the body works and what it needs to heal, I believe his life was cut short.

A RETURN TO HEALTH

So what can you do to get your health back? Start by accepting that degenerative diseases are almost the sole result of our poor lifestyle and food choices. Responsibility is the first place to turn to if we want lasting results. One can do many things to prevent diseases, but we just aren't doing them, many times out of ignorance.

For example, I think that most people underestimate the tremendous benefits of exercise. According to the Centers for Disease Control and Prevention (CDC) people who participate in 7 hours of physical activity per week have a 40% lower risk of premature death than those who participate in less than 30 minutes per week.[14] Adding a daily exercise routine to your schedule is the one thing that you can do that will contribute to a large range of benefits, from helping to prevent illness to increased energy and better restorative sleep to adding more fun and excitement to your life! On the other hand living a sedentary lifestyle has as many and even more far-reaching, impactful, negative consequences. The CDC lists the following benefits of physical activity:

- Controls your weight
- Reduces your risk of cardiovascular disease
- Reduces your risk of type 2 diabetes and metabolic syndrome
- Reduces your risk of some cancers
- Strengthens your bones and muscles
- Improves your mental health and mood
- Improves your ability to do daily activities and prevent falls, if you're an older adult
- Increases your chances of living longer

Once you start eating what your body needs, not what you feel like eating, and get into a routine of some daily physical activity, you will begin to feel immediate positive changes.

If you are struggling to eat healthily or if it seems like too much of an effort, you may be dealing with an addiction to certain foods like wheat, dairy or sweet foods. These can be difficult addictions to break. Get some help. There are programs out there that help break refined, high glycemic, carbohydrate addictions. If you really desire to make these changes but you keep slipping back, or if it seems too overwhelming, you may also want to look at the emotional and unconscious part of you that may be sabotaging your health efforts. We look more in-depth concerning these issues in the next chapter. There are also many holistic therapists that can aid you in establishing healthy eating habits.

Hopefully you are now convinced that when we consume a lot of packaged, canned, processed foods or fast foods which are filled with all kinds of additives, we not only become undernourished but we also build up chemicals and other toxic substances in our bodies. The body tries to evacuate these substances, but if they keep coming in with no respite, and if our eliminating organs are not working so well, the body will begin to hide these toxins to get them out of circulation. The liver may signal fat cells to store these toxins and this makes it even more difficult to lose weight. In addition, acidic toxic substances, stress and unhealthy lifestyle create free radicals which irritate and damage our tissues and cells, which produces inflammation inside our bodies and leads to all kinds of degenerative diseases.

CHRONIC SYSTEMIC INFLAMMATION

Chronic systemic inflammation is epidemic in our society today. The danger of this type of inflammation is that it is continually in operation and it is silent. When inflammation takes place deep inside the body, we are not able to feel any pain and we can't see any signs like redness or swelling. We therefore cannot proactively respond to the damage it is causing inside our body. Our immune system, however, does respond to this inflammation, but in the process of this response it also destroys our good cells and tissue, creating all kinds of autoimmune disorders. In fact, chronic inflammation is linked to almost every degenerative disease. The problem is that we don't even know it's there, silently destroying our body, often until it's too late.

Lyle MacWilliam, a biochemist and author of *The Nutritional Guide to Supplements*, explains that increased amounts of insulin in our blood – whether it be from a high sugar consumption, the beginnings of insulin resistance, or the hormonal effect of excess fat – lays the groundwork for systemic inflammation. However, it's the consequences of the unhealthy North American diet, rich in pro-inflammatory omega 6 fatty acids and low in anti-inflammatory omega 3 fatty acids, that is resulting in systemic inflammation.[15] The body releases cortisol in response to this inflammation. However, while trying to reduce inflammation, cortisol also raises blood pressure and triggers the release of more glucose in the blood, which then increases the production of insulin. This creates a vicious cycle of continued inflammation, which creates more and more cellular damage, leading to all kinds of diseases including heart disease and cancer. Systemic inflammation is a silent killer.

Many other lifestyle choices also contribute to this kind of inflammation, such as smoking, obesity, chronic stress and drinking alcohol in excess. Fortunately, these negative factors can be changed. As we reduce inflammation by making positive lifestyle changes today, we will decrease the risks of dying from cancer or other degenerative diseases tomorrow.

> SILENT CHRONIC INFLAMMATION COMES FROM AN IMBALANCE BETWEEN OMEGA 6 FATTY ACIDS AND OMEGA 3 FATTY ACIDS

A QUESTION TO MEDICAL SCIENCE

With all the recent medical advancements, why has medical science not found remedies for these rampant degenerative diseases? Could it be that a great contributor to the source of the problem of degenerative diseases is what we eat or don't eat, and what we are exposed to in the form of toxic chemicals? Could it be that our unhealthy, stressful lifestyles are also contributing to our malaise? In addition, could the lack of daily physical exercise impede the functioning of our detoxification organs that help remove toxins from our body? Maybe we're seeing the wrong professionals to get help for these kinds of diseases.

Doctors are trained to diagnose disease, treat symptoms and intervene in emergencies. When it comes to disease prevention, doctors are not necessarily the experts we need to be confiding in. If we want to live a healthy, disease-free life, it is essential we intervene long before a disease can be detected by lab tests or medical equipment. Let's put ourselves on the offensive by practising preventive medicine.

We can train ourselves to begin listening to the early warning signals our body is giving us and not wait until sickness is detected through medical diagnostics before starting to do something to get healthier. It's easy to ignore the early signals. We are busy, focused on other things. It's true that we have not necessarily been taught how to notice these small warning signs and therefore are simply not in the habit of doing so. Perhaps it's also because we may have relinquished the responsibility of our health to the medical profession, thinking they hold all of the answers regarding our health. We must take responsibility by taking proactive steps towards restoring and maintaining our own health.

Degenerative diseases do not overtake us out of the blue. They mostly appear because of our chronic detrimental lifestyle habits. Many diseases are really not that complicated to heal, especially if we start addressing the problem in the initial stages of dis-ease. I realize that training ourselves to eat differently, to listen to our bodies as well as noticing and then changing our negative thought patterns can be a challenge, especially if we have never done this before. There are all kinds of alternative health practitioners that can assist you to help rectify your eating and lifestyle habits. Others can help assist you in identifying symptoms that could possibly lead to future illnesses that at this stage would not yet be detectable through medical diagnostics. Coaches, counsellors or therapists can assist you with stress, negative emotions and negative thought patterns. In chapter 7, I have included a short list of alternative health professions that you may refer to. Take advantage of their support to help you turn things around.

THERMOGRAPHY AND MAMMOGRAMS

Breast Thermography is not a diagnostic tool but rather a type of screening tool that helps detect the earliest possible signs of breast cancer even before they show up on a mammogram. Cancerous cells necessitate new blood vessel formation for their survival. This causes an increase in blood flow, which in turn causes an increase in temperature in the affected area. This temperature increase can be detected by thermal analysis when the duplication of cancer cells is still at its beginnings. Early detection is the key to breast cancer survival rate. Mammograms, on the other hand, can only detect cancer cells after they have been developing over the course of several years. A "normal" mammogram result does not necessarily mean no cancer. Mammograms, in addition to being very uncomfortable and sometimes painful, use radiation, which is known to cause cancer in certain cases.[16] Non-invasive, non-radioactive thermography can be used to detect abnormal activity, which can then be used in conjunction with other conventional diagnostic tests to confirm the presence of cancer. You then have the opportunity to change your diet and lifestyle, empowering your body to be in a better position in order to overcome the cancer in its initial stages.

CONSEQUENCES FOR FUTURE GENERATIONS

Did you know that some babies are being born with certain degenerative diseases? They come into the world affected with diabetes, childhood lymphomas, brain tumours and other such diseases. This is sad and must be overwhelming for parents. A study conducted with the Environmental Working Group in cooperation with the American Red Cross looked at the umbilical cords from newborns and found, on average, 200 toxic industrial compounds. More than 180 of them were carcinogenic, or cancer causing, in humans or animals.[17]

If women of childbearing age have cellular terrain that is unhealthy because of poor eating habits and constant exposure to chemicals in their home living environment, they risk affecting the health of their future babies. It is of utmost importance for pregnant women to eat healthily and to reinforce their immune system and that of their growing baby through an optimal dietary regime, but also to be very vigilant as to the toxins present in the air surrounding them – especially those found in their own homes.

Pregnant women and nursing mothers unknowingly expose their babies to chemical residues from hair sprays, dry-cleaning fluids, perfumes, toilet deodorizers, and other household and personal care products that they are using. These chemicals can be unsafe for a growing baby, especially during the gestation period. Even though there is a possibility of passing on these chemicals through breast milk, there is a much greater impact with the baby's own exposure to airborne pollutants. Young babies' fragile and still developing organs and immune systems are much more vulnerable to the ill effects of these chemical scents than we can imagine. It is therefore highly recommended that women become aware of and reduce exposure to these products in order to reduce the associated risks.[18]

Men are no exception to this situation. We've seen the research indicating how exposure to environmental chemicals has caused low sperm count and other infertility problems. If the fertility health of the father is in jeopardy, how can that not impact the quality of genes being passed down to the offspring? It is best when men as well as women are the healthiest they can be before planning to conceive a child. A three-month preconception detox program would be very beneficial for both – and for baby too! A six-month program or more would be even better.

In order to bring about beneficial change in our health status, it is essential that we start asking ourselves how our actions and food choices adversely affect our good health and not just let ourselves be influenced by the masses, nonchalantly eating whatever is before us. Hence the importance of being pro-active and committed. The impact of our being negligent in our nutritional habits and lifestyle choices has a potentially far-reaching negative consequence not only on us and our children, but also on our children's children. Without our realizing it, we may be contributing to the diseases of our future generations through the small, seemingly insignificant, poor choices we make today. We are doing this both by example and by passing down our subsequently less-than-optimal, chemically altered genes.

Our examples speak loudly. What we say to our kids will never have a greater impact than what they see us doing or not doing. Our actions will naturally get passed down, much more so than any intellectual teaching, especially if what we teach is not congruent with our actions. For example, we can't say: "Don't eat candy; it's not good for you," all the while eating sugar coated doughnuts or eating processed, sweetened, packaged breakfast cereals. We humans learn more by example than by cognition. Let's make an effort to change our lifestyle choices for the benefit of our children's future as well as our own.

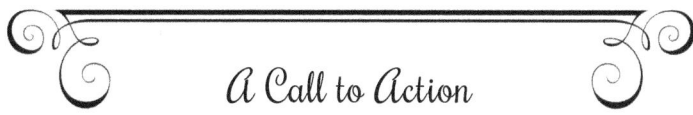

A Call to Action

How about you? Are you living with some degenerative disease? Have you lived your life's purpose? If you left this earth before your time, would there be people who will have missed out on what you could have brought them? Can you leave this world with a sense of having lived your dreams and walked into your destiny? If not, please, I urgently encourage you to consider these things. If your red dashboard lights are flickering, your body is giving you signs. Find out why and start making some positive healthy changes. Find an alternative healthcare practitioner or other healthcare consultant qualified to help you get to the root cause of your ailments. Take charge of your health and put into action the steps that will give you a revitalized, healthy body so that you can live the life you were meant to live and walk in the destiny you were created to walk in.

SUMMARY

- **There is something you can do to reverse cancer and other degenerative diseases.** You can do even more to prevent them. Your body is equipped with a dashboard that informs you when things are going awry. Learning to listen to and interpreting these indicators, as well as beginning to make adjustments right from the start, can prevent the development of disease.

- **The good news has to get out: food does heal.** God has provided us with whole foods from nature to help us thrive and be healthy. He has provided in nature the elements necessary to help us heal. It's the miracle cure we are all looking for.

- **When faced with cancer or any other degenerative disease, eating and lifestyle become part of a whole different ballgame.** You cannot continue to eat what you have always been eating. The neutral pH of your body has drastically changed to an acidic one. You, therefore, need to be on the offensive to help your body heal by eating healthier alkaline foods. Yes, it's a radical change, but it greatly contributes to combatting acidity and inflammation, which helps bring about healing.

- **There is a real emotional aspect to all disease.** Cancer patients especially profit from the loving support of their close ones, accompanied by pertinent professional help to be able to make these often difficult changes in their lives, as well as working through those buried, unspoken negative emotions. It is also essential that they begin to love themselves unconditionally.

- **You have nothing to lose by trying.** I know that not all cancers or other diseases will be totally healed by making these healthy lifestyle changes. If a person is seriously ill and doesn't heal, taking an offensive approach and making those beneficial changes to their diet and lifestyle can give them a greater quality of life and make a significant difference in the way that they live the last part of their life.

- **Awareness can change your life.** The most important steps that you can take to prevent degenerative diseases and cancer are to be more aware of and reduce your chemical exposure, both to chemicals created inside your body through stressful, negative emotions and those chemicals coming from outside your body – mainly from your own home environment. Additionally, if you can understand how food and nutrition play a vital role in healing, you can start making even small steps towards changing what you consume. As you do this, as well as including a daily physical fitness program, you will develop a body that is more resilient and more resistant to disease.

Much of our daily routine is habitual, and we all know how difficult it can be to change that, even if it isn't really working for us. The good news is, if we can learn negative habits, we can also learn positive ones. In the following chapter we'll identify a few more items that need to be addressed, allowing you to be even more pro-active in your journey to health and healing.

5
CHAPTER FIVE

A radical change towards good health

Now that we better understand that many diseases stem from an unhealthy lifestyle, poor diet, chronic stress and strong negative emotions, in addition to inadequate detoxification, the next step forward is to ask ourselves what we can do to change things around. Many of us, especially those over 40, may be under the impression that because most of our peers suffer from some kind of pain or disease, that this is a natural part of the aging process. Additionally, because we lack awareness of the true nature of our diseases, and because of our ignorance to the negative impact of repetitively making bad choices, we have given in to the creation of bad habits. When sickness manifests we turn to medication, which more often than not is a temporary solution to a much deeper problem.

When we look more closely at our diets and lifestyles, it becomes evident that the source of this sudden increase in disease has to do with our collective addiction to processed, nutritionally deficient foods. This cultural blindness has been spurred on by a corporate food industry that markets unnatural foods laden with toxic additives as "wholesome" and "healthy". Moreover, we tend to overlook how our deep-rooted negative beliefs about ourselves may be sabotaging our efforts or motivation to change what we can. This keeps us spinning our wheels in frustration and despair, perhaps even causing us to throw in the towel, giving up any effort to do anything differently. However, once we realize how much unhealthy food we are in fact consuming, and as we begin to listen to our body and acknowledge our unconscious negative beliefs, we may begin the journey to establishing longstanding good health for ourselves, our families and our communities.

IGNORANCE IS – A TEMPORARY – BLISS

Lack of knowledge is a huge reason why many people end up falling sick and remaining sick. One cannot escape the physical laws that pertain to having a healthy body. In fact, we can deduce many of the principles that support these natural laws, based on logic and common sense. Unfortunately, common sense and logic have been pushed further and further from our reach in our new modern era of fast food and packaged, processed products taking over our food markets. Stop and think for an instant: it makes sense that if we eat more whole foods and fewer processed foods, our body will perform better.

If we cannot distinguish between whole and processed foods to ensure better health, we not only unnecessarily expose ourselves to disease but we also risk passing on this lack of common sense to the next generation. They will have no benchmarks to measure against to see if a food is good or not. Many children do not eat the minimum daily requirement of 400 grams of fruits and vegetables recommended by the WHO (World Health Organization).[1] If you include a serving of potatoes (or hash browns or French fries) in this number, this will leave room for approximately one banana and one apple. It is evident that children are not being exposed to a large variety of vegetables and fruits, making some of them unable to tell the difference between a whole food like an apple and processed food like a packaged breakfast cereal. Vegetables, other than the basic tomato and lettuce, are often foreign to them.

Reacquainting ourselves with real whole food and the basic laws of healthy eating is vital to making sure that we maintain healthy bodies for ourselves and for our children. The problem is that the food industry has assaulted us with propaganda that has tricked this generation into thinking that coloured stuff in a box or anything pre-packaged is real, nourishing food. It's also true for those of us who grew up with real foods. We are also being lead to believe that we are eating something nutritionally good for us because it says on the box "fortified with iron", or marks the addition of some vitamin, mineral or other faddish expression. Let's start questioning our automatic (perhaps naïve), unhealthy lifestyle choices and return to using common sense, coupled with a cause and effect reflection. Becoming informed helps, so in the next chapters we will be covering basic principles and steps that will help you understand what is required in order to be healthy.

HABITS AND OUR LIFESTYLE CHOICES

You have heard the saying, "Habits make or break us." It holds true in the area of our food intake also. Most of us eat whatever seems to catch our eye or whatever we are most in the habit of eating. Unfortunately, many of these foods tend to be refined foods, mostly void of nutritional value. Additionally, many people often drink soda pop or fruit juices with their meals – it's just a habit. Not only are these beverages not healthy for us (for reasons we will come to shortly), but drinking while we eat dilutes our enzymes thereby decreasing the capacity for our food to get digested properly.

How about having a nice, sugary dessert right after your meals? It may seem inconceivable, but once you start eating well and as your body becomes more balanced, you can get out of that habit, too. Eating sugary deserts after your meals may actually start fermenting the food already in your stomach, causing digestive problems. Besides, we all know that refined sugar is not good for us.

THE MANY DRAWBACKS OF HIGH SUGAR CONSUMPTION

Americans consume on average 94 grams of sugar per day, or approximately 76 pounds of sugar per year.[2] Even though this amount has slightly decreased since the 1999 all-time high, that's still a lot of sugar to be consuming. We may not be aware of the actual amounts of sugar we really do consume, because refined sugar is hidden in many processed foods. Every time we eat sugary foods our immune system becomes suppressed. Another detrimental fact that we tend not to realize is that processed carbohydrates – anything that is made with white flour, for example – act like sugar in the body. That's one reason why it's smart not to consume sweets or refined carbohydrates like bagels, doughnuts, cookies, etc., especially when we are fighting a cold, flu or any other illness. That's also why many people fall sick during holidays like Christmas and Easter: the increased consumption of cakes, cookies and other sweets does not permit the immune system to fight back properly.

Eating these kinds of foods fills us up with empty calories and increases our appetites because our cells communicate to our body that they are still hungry. They have not been nourished with the good nutrition that cells require to operate properly. Weight gain and poor health become consequences of too much sugar or refined carbohydrate consumption. Replacing sweet foods with fresh fruits, vegetables, good, healthy fats and good-quality protein will do the exact opposite.

In chapter 4 we saw how high sugar intake lays the groundwork for inflammation in our bodies, and how chronic systemic inflammation is the precursor to most degenerative diseases. Regularly consuming refined white flour products or sugar also causes us to age faster. In chapter 2, we discovered how the formation of AGEs (Advanced Glycation End products) due to a diet high in sugar, irritates cells, causing tissue damage, inflammation and premature aging. The more sugar you eat, the higher the production of AGEs, and the higher the risk for degenerative diseases like diabetes, Alzheimer's and heart disease. High sugar consumption also causes loss of elasticity in your skin, not to mention an increase in insulin. Chronically high insulin not only causes weight gain and high blood pressure, but also contributes to premature aging.

THE DANGERS OF HIGH FRUCTOSE CORN SYRUP

High fructose corn syrup (HFCS) is the primary sweetener used in many U.S. soft drinks and is in many fruit beverages. HFCS is cheaper and sweeter than sucrose (table sugar). This explains why food and beverage manufacturers have turned to its broad usage. This dangerous sweetener is not only found in soft drinks but in all kinds of processed foods like cookies, baked goods, jams and jellies, salad dressings and in many beverages such as fruit juices and fruit drinks.

Fructose is dangerous because it does not get digested the way other sugars do. Once consumed, it goes directly to your liver to get metabolized.[3] In the liver, the fructose gets turned into fats such as triglycerides and VLDL (very "bad") cholesterol. High levels of these kinds of fats lead to heart disease and non-alcoholic fatty liver disease. When you consume food that contains HFCS your appetite actually increases because your satiation hormone, leptin, does not get triggered, letting you know you have eaten enough. It is a great contributing cause to the obesity epidemic.

The process of metabolising fructose by your liver also creates waste products such as uric acid, which causes gout and can also cause high blood pressure.

High fructose corn syrup causes many health problems and is not something that you want to be consuming. To protect yourself, be an avid label verifier and eliminate the consumption of fruit juices and fruit beverages. Fructose found in fresh fruit does not contribute to this kind of problem because of the fibre and other phytonutrients present in whole fruit. However, depending on your health situation, you may want to keep your fruit consumption to a moderate to low level.

Coming back to our lifestyle and habits, let's consider, for instance, the habit of drinking a "good" cup of coffee (or two) in the morning. This habit may get you revved up and awake to start the day. But it's not the revving up that you need if you want to keep your body alkaline or if you don't want to contribute to adrenal burnout due to excess amounts of cortisol flooding your system. Yes, it's true that caffeine makes your thoughts more clear and you feel more awake. But this is because coffee has triggered your body to produce the stress hormones adrenaline and cortisol. Habitual drinks like coffee should be used in moderation and should be organic (free of chemicals) if at all possible. If you are suffering from burnout – adrenal fatigue – or you are going through a period of prolonged stress, coffee should be avoided all together.

Another example of a tenacious bad habit is that we tend to eat late at night or sometimes just before going to bed. It's at this time that our body is slowing down its digestive functions in order to focus more on the restoring, rebuilding and detoxification that it will soon be doing while we sleep. If we consume food in the later evening, our digestive system doesn't get a chance to restore completely. It will be busy digesting. During the day, our metabolism is focused on providing us with energy through this laborious digestion process. Consequently, there is not adequate restoration or rebuilding of the body. That's why our metabolism concentrates on these tasks at night while we are sleeping and the body is at rest. Did you know that children actually grow at night and not during the day for the very same reason? That's why it's so important to allow our body to do its crucial nightly regenerative tasks without interruption.

To sum up, when the body is forced to digest food late at night, it delays the rebuilding, restoration and waste removal cycle. We then wake up feeling groggy and not totally refreshed. This unfavourable late night eating habit may create a vicious cycle where we need that cup of coffee to get us going in the morning!

There are other benefits of not eating in the evening. The time in which our body is fasting is extended – when we sleep, we are actually fasting – which naturally assists in weight management.

There are many other little seemingly inoffensive habits that gradually contribute to illness: not chewing our food adequately, eating junk food way too often or indulging in lots of quick, easy-to-prepare processed, packaged foods, being too busy to partake in regular exercise, not being exposed to enough sunlight and fresh air, not ensuring that we are getting enough good quality sleep, being addicted to stress, not drinking enough pure water and not eating enough green vegetables. I am not talking about being perfect. It's not that piece of birthday cake that we indulge in once in a while that will bring eventually devastating results, but rather it's the cumulative effect of what we do every day adding up over a lifetime.

DIET, LIFESTYLE AND THE CHALLENGES OF MENOPAUSE

At a certain age, women will enter into a new phase of life that will gradually evolve into the cessation of fertility, called menopause. Although this is a very natural part of life and all women are destined to go through this, it can be a very challenging time for many. The transition into menopause – whether difficult or smooth – will be determined greatly by the sum of our experiences and habits, good or bad, up until this point in our lives. If we are not living an overly stressful life, have had good, healthy eating habits, have partaken in regular exercise, and we have a positive outlook on life, not having allowed bitterness, disillusionment or dissatisfaction to accumulate as well as having allowed the healing of our inner emotional wounds to take place, the transition will be easier.

Life happens, and perhaps – because we have been so busy or because we have not had the right tools to help us face hurts, pain or any other difficult circumstances that we may have come across – we may have let these issues go unprocessed. This is a time where we are given another chance to address and resolve any emotional difficulties we have not dealt with up until now. Menopause is a time when our body is going though many changes, which in itself is a challenge. It's also a time when our body is letting us know that what we have pushed under the carpet can no longer be left unattended. Emotional health affects physical health. Normal hormonal changes in menopause causes symptoms like night sweats, hot flashes, brain fog and mood changes, but these can be exacerbated by stress and strong, negative, un-dealt with emotions. Be vigilant to take care of your emotional health. Uncovering and facing these feelings will help make this transition much easier. I encourage women who are going through this stage in life to take advantage of this passage to address any of these uncomfortable, un-dealt with issues. This frees you up to courageously go forward into the next adventurous season of your life. Make sure to surround yourself with supportive relationships; it is essential for your wellbeing.

Unhealthy dietary habits like high consumption of refined carbohydrates, or sugary foods and drinking coffee or alcohol can also contribute to more intense menopausal symptoms. The correct hormonal balance is also vital to a woman's health. If you are going through a challenging time in this season of your life, it would be beneficial to get your hormones checked. Safe, natural approaches can often be used to correct imbalances.

THE HIGH RETURNS OF BEING PROACTIVE

We eat almost anything we want, whenever we want, never thinking that there can be any serious consequence or connection between what goes into our mouth and the state of our health. We get used to eating certain foods and don't even question whether they are good for us or not. Basically, we eat whatever is being catered to us.

We eat the food that big business produces. For instance, when we go to a restaurant, the menu determines what we can eat. Our choice will often be based on or influenced by how the food tastes and not necessarily on what nutritional value the food will bring to our cells. Processed foods and the majority of restaurant foods are loaded with invisible ingredients to make the food taste good. We know that these foods contain an overabundance of salt, sugar, MSG (mono sodium glutamate) and most likely GMO food and trans fats (although more and more laws are now lowering and even restricting the use of trans fats in restaurants). Not only do we give little thought as to whether the food we eat contributes to our wellbeing, we have also lost confidence in our ability to inherently know what is good for us or what is not. We regularly eat the food that causes many of our maladies.

To control the quality of the food that we ingest, we can cook more wholesome meals at home. Restaurant food, in general, could be reserved for special occasions, unless you know for certain the high quality of the food being served. If your job or life situation does not permit you to cook your own healthy meals at home on a regular basis, you can take control of your health even in a restaurant by ordering foods that are healthier for you, even if they are not necessarily listed on the menu. For example, instead of fries, ask for a baked potato and eat the peel as well for extra fibre, or exchange the white rice for a steamed vegetable or extra salad. However, if you eat in restaurants daily, with the exception of certain specific, health-conscious restaurants, you, more than anyone else, need to follow some detox program several times per year, as well as ensuring you add supplements to your diet daily.

> **THERE IS A CONNECTION BETWEEN WHAT GOES INTO OUR MOUTH AND THE STATE OF OUR HEALTH**

If you want to be preventive in your approach, you must not wait until you have aches and pains that are so intense that you urgently need to see a doctor. Learn to listen to the small warning signals or symptoms your body emits early on. Notice if there is a connection with what you are eating, to the stress or emotions that you are experiencing, or to other environmental factors to which you are exposed.

Often times when we are in pain and because we have tuned out those small early signals, fear sets in and we hurriedly rush to the doctor for help. Perhaps with a bit of reflection we could have determined the cause and effect ourselves and then made healthy adjustments. It's our responsibility to tune in and try and find the connection. If we neglect to do this, then it warrants a visit to the doctor's office in order to help us diagnose what is wrong. Also realize that even though most medical doctors sincerely want to help their patients, they will do so from their perspective, using their pharmaceutical expertise. They will most probably prescribe you medication. Even though taking medication may give you temporary relief, it will also shut down your red warning lights. If you are not simultaneously treating the root cause and making some dietary or lifestyle changes, it will only be a matter of time before another red warning light pops up. Dealing with the root issue can not only get rid of your symptom, it can eliminate the problem at its source.

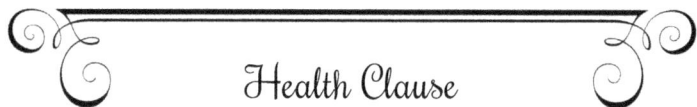

Health Clause

Note: if you have been struggling with some health issues for some time and have neglected to address the symptoms, the situation may have become too advanced to simply resort to preventive measures. It is your responsibility to go for a medical check-up in order to better assess what you are dealing with. Don't hesitate to get a second opinion from another doctor if necessary.

I encourage you to also seek the advice of an alternative health professional for alternative non-invasive treatments. Evaluate both conventional and alternative recommendation and weigh the potential negative and positive consequences to both approaches. In many cases, following the recommendations of an alternative health specialist will help you treat the root cause of your malaise. Regardless of the direction you take, you are the person responsible for the health solutions you choose. Furthermore, I encourage you to do your own research and to not let fear dictate your decisions.

ANTIBIOTICS

Antibiotics are used to treat overgrowth of bad bacteria. However, over the years there has been an overuse and misuse of antibiotics. They have wrongly been prescribed to treat viral infections. This often happens when a patient goes to the doctor because of a sore throat and is looking for immediate relief. The doctor may prescribe antibiotics just in case it is a bacterial infection, like strep throat for example. A swab test may be taken, but the problem is that it may take several days for the lab results to come back. The patient often does not want to wait that long and so begins to take the prescription immediately. This misuse contributes to antibiotic resistance. Additionally, the patient who does not respect the dosage or the duration of the treatment may permit the bacteria to survive also causing the bacteria to become resistant. The challenge with antibiotic resistance is that common but more serious infections such as pneumonia or cystitis (urine infection) may no longer respond to antibiotics, putting at risk the lives of patients.

Viral infections, like the common cold and influenza, cannot be treated with antibiotics. Even though no one appreciates having a cold or the flu, they rarely cause serious harm. These are simply ailments that need to run their course, usually lasting from 7 to 10 days and sometimes up to 3 weeks. Rest and lots of liquids are called for during these times. A well-balanced diet, including fruits and vegetables, also helps boost your immune system.

Common side effects of almost all antibiotics are stomach problems such as abdominal cramps, gas, nausea, vomiting and diarrhoea. This is because the antibiotics used to destroy disease-causing bacteria in your respiratory tract (your throat or sinuses for example) also destroy good gut bacteria. This bacterial disequilibrium disrupts your digestive health and may cause the appearance of *Candida albicans* (thrush) or the overgrowth of other bacteria such as *C. difficile* (Clostridium difficile). Whenever taking antibiotics, and it should be only when it is absolutely necessary, simultaneously taking a pro-biotic (good bacteria) supplement or eating fermented foods can prevent these undesirable gastrointestinal side effects from happening.

A QUESTION OF DISCIPLINE

"Eat to live, not live to eat". What a great adage! My friends, this takes a lot of determination and the retraining of our habits and negative lifestyle choices. But hey, you are worth it aren't you? The responsibility for your health is on your shoulders. I encourage you to do some research to try and figure out why you are getting sick and find out what makes your body feel good and revitalized. It is also of importance to attend alternative health seminars and workshops, and invest in the reading of books pertaining to this subject. Understanding gained through information gathering, examples and testimonies keeps us motivated.

Because we are being bombarded with so much propaganda and advertising of wrong food consumption, we have to consciously rethink and reconsider everything we put into our mouths. Find a health coach, a naturopath or another alternative health practitioner. They can inform and assist you in deducing what is good for you and what is not. This can be a remarkable way to support you in changing your lifestyle and tenacious bad habits one step at a time. This is also a great way to keep you accountable, helping to ensure positive results.

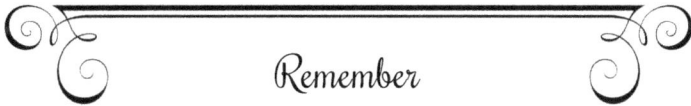

It's not about what you can't eat, but what your body needs to heal and be healthy.

PHYSICAL ACTIVITY

Being physically active is another initiative that we will want to act on in our pursuit of great health. It's one of the very important factors to having optimal health and a resilient body. Remember, living a sedentary lifestyle is one of the 5 major contributing factors that leads to degenerative diseases. It is crucial to implement regular physical activity into our schedule. Yes it does take an act of our will to do the things that in the moment may feel like a lot of effort. In time this discipline will bring us freedom and confidence to engage in whatever life activities that we choose, even as we grow older.

Establishing the habit of participating in physical activities starts in early age. That is why it is so very important to ensure that our young children are active, playing outdoors and participating in different physical activities or programs as they grow. It's very easy for children to become sedentary because they can spend a lot of time in front of some type of screen – computer, TV or other. It is crucial for children to stimulate their cardiac output and oxygenate their cells with energetic physical movement. Developing this habit at a young age will help contribute to an active lifestyle later on. I encourage you to think proactively for your children, especially beginning at a young age, and create or find fun physical activities and events in which they can participate regularly, even if it's playing tag in the park.

Without exercise our muscles become sluggish and weak. A consistent fitness program, as well as proper nutrition, builds our muscles and can even reverse the muscle loss that accompanies old age. Again, this all starts with taking personal responsibility for our health. It is wise to initiate this habit early in life, but remember that whatever your age, it's never too late to begin.

Engrained bad habits are created by repetitive action over time; engrained good habits are created in the same manner. Discipline is the master to be called upon when we want to make sure we integrate these positive changes. To make it easier to stick to an exercise routine, choose a physical activity you enjoy and do it from a perspective of love, of you wanting to do good to you. This brings pleasure, and also gives us vibrant energy and vitality. Fitness (or physical activity) energizes us, makes us feel and look good, and, as previously mentioned by the CDC, lowers the risk for developing degenerative disease. It can also help with chronic pain, depression and is a great way to alleviate stress.

Lack of physical activity has many detrimental consequences including a listless, frail, weak, toxic body. I encourage you, whatever your age, young or old, to do everything that you can to initiate and maintain some kind of fitness program. Doing so will help you age with strength and vitality and not let the problems of a weak body interfere with living your life to the fullest. Let's face it: it is easier to deal with obstacles of any kind when we have a strong, healthy body.

If we think of our body as our partner, or our "buddy", we can literally ask our buddy what it needs today. Say to yourself, "Hey, bud, what can I do for you today?" And then, of course, if we love our buddy, we will first listen and then give it what it needs. In turn it can love us back and do what it can to give us good – even great – health so that we may fulfill our dreams, walk in our potential, and experience our destiny. How powerful is that? It is a love relationship with our body – our buddy.

If we don't love our buddy by attentively giving it what it needs, we will eat whatever we feel like eating, caring only to stimulate our taste buds and fill our stomach and procrastinate when it comes to doing our physical exercises. Our time and energy will be spent on pondering how much effort it takes to get up and get going instead of actually doing the exercises.

Tuning into what really nourishes us, including the physical movement our body desperately needs, will help our body perform at its best.

ADDICTED TO PROCESSED FOODS

Finally, I believe our society is dealing with a chronic addiction to bad food. A 2015 Weight Watchers® advertisement that I retrieved on YouTube featured an ironic adaptation of the musical tune "If You're Happy and You Know It", which demonstrates this perfectly.[4] It goes like this:

If you're happy and you know it, eat a snack.

If you're happy and you know it, eat a snack.

If you're happy and you know it, then your face will surely show it.

If you're happy and you know it, eat a snack.

If you're sad and you know it, eat a snack.

If you're sad and you know it, eat a snack.

If you're sad because you're angry, feeling down or generally bad,

If you're sad, eat a snack.

If you're bored and you know it, eat a snack.

If you're lonely and you know it, eat a snack.

If you're sleepy and you know it,

If you're guilty and you know it,

If you're stressed, eat a snack.

If you're human and you know it, then your face will surely show it.

If you're human, eat your feelings. Eat a snack.

The video clip that goes with the song depicts this even better. Let me list the snack foods presented in the video:

- Ice-cream
- Cake
- Pop
- Hamburger
- Pizza
- Chocolate bar

- Doritos® chips with melted Cheez Whiz®
- Buttered popcorn
- Potato chips
- More ice-cream
- More cake
- White-bread sandwich
- Candy
- Nachos
- Pogo

Folks, these "snacks" are the food products that are killing us, and we are eating way too many of them. They have become our everyday staple food. I'm not saying that we should never eat these food products. Some committed, passionate health advocates don't, and the more power to them. But for the most part, I don't think that the whole of society can become that fervent. However, I do believe that we all can begin to take small steps forward to gain our health back. These processed foods need to be treated as festive foods, "treats" that we eat only once in a while.

We strongly resist passing up or exchanging these unhealthy foods for more healthy, real foods like vegetables and fruits. We tend to think that our life wouldn't be complete without processed treats, or that we might not survive without them. In fact, we are unknowingly and literally dying for them. I don't think many of us will say on our death beds: "I wish I had eaten more ice-cream sundaes or more potato chips or drank more soft drinks or eaten more French fries and hamburgers." No, I rather think we would say: "I wish I would have developed my gifts, had more close relationships and lived my life with intentionality and purpose." Unhealthy processed foods as well as lack of physical exercise stops us from developing our full potential. We become lethargic and lack energy. We numb ourselves with food. We sabotage our lives and our destiny with food. Our unhealthy lifestyle choices are killing us slowly but surely.

If you are fighting a life-threatening disease – whether it be obesity, diabetes, heart disease or cancer – and you want to have a fighting chance to recuperate, then processed foods absolutely need to be completely eliminated from your diet. It takes discipline to make the right choices and self-love to sustain this effort. You will find that initiating new habits, and persevering until they become second nature, is well worth the effort. Overcoming these food addictions requires a lot of determination, but it is possible. Get the support you need.

Right from the start, young children should not be exposed to eating processed foods on a regular basis. We need to help children develop their taste buds for real food while they are still young so that they don't develop these unhealthy addictions at an early age. This way the building blocks (their cells) for their future adult bodies will be strong and resistant to disease. They will have developed the habit of eating well. They will know what real food is. Then they can be permitted to eat a bit of these processed foods on occasion.

Let's face it, these processed foods are not going away. We have to learn to live with them, so I suggest that we get a handle on these types of foods and that we make them rare, occasional foods. Restricting our kids and disciplining ourselves from eating these foods on an everyday basis is imperative.

We can compare being addicted to processed foods to alcoholism. Once you have recovered from alcohol abuse and try to take one small drink, the desire to drink more will have a good chance of overtaking you. So you have to abstain. If you are already addicted to these food products you can change things around. Start to add in ample amounts of vitamin-and mineral-dense whole foods, such as raw vegetables and some fruits, as well as a lot of good healthy fats and some healthy proteins. As a result, you will slowly be replacing harmful food with nutritious food. You may need to get some help and support to make these changes; don't be reluctant to do so. If you do so consistently and for a long enough period of time, gradually building a strong foundation of regularly eating healthy foods, you will tilt the scales to the positive and will then be able to manage the occasional indulgence without being thrown back in the addiction camp and not being able to resist any kind of temptation.

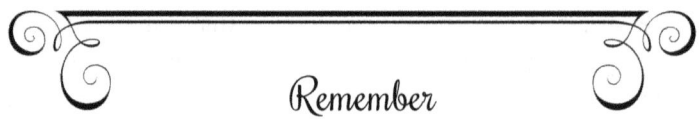

Moderation is always in good taste.

LOW SELF-ESTEEM:
UNCONSCIOUS NEGATIVE BELIEFS ABOUT ONESELF

So far we have looked at 4 major factors that contribute to the development of disease: nutrient deficiency, overload of toxins, stress and negative emotions and sedentary lifestyle. The 5th contributing factor is our self-image or our unconscious negative belief system. It's subtle, but it can be the root cause of our sickness, undermining our capacity to make good choices for our health.

The first few years of our lives are critical and can have a positive as well as a negative impact on us. Psychologists say that usually before the age of six we have already determined what life will be like for us. For many of us, regardless of our early childhood experiences, this tends to include a negative self-image. Often, these erroneous conclusions that we have made of ourselves, even though done unconsciously and at a very young age, will be the basis on which we will determine our value for the rest of our lives, if of course we do nothing to reprogram them.

Reflecting on how we value ourselves is something we may want to explore if we want to put all the odds on our side for having a healthier life. For instance, some of our negative addictions to food, as well as our self-sabotaging mechanisms in the area of our health, can be propelled by unresolved negative, unconscious beliefs about ourselves. If we think we are not worthy, we unconsciously act in a way that leads us to wrong eating and to not being interested or motivated in making that extra effort to do the things that will help us get back on track to a healthy lifestyle. We consequently live in denial, covering up by making excuses and justifying why it is impossible for us to make certain necessary lifestyle and dietary changes. If we unconsciously don't feel good about ourselves, we tend to unknowingly sabotage our efforts to eat well.

Often times we use unhealthy foods to make us feel better. Anyone who has tried to go on a diet has had to face the temptation of consuming certain kinds of problem foods that should be avoided. These comfort foods consist mainly of processed carbohydrates, which are also high-glycemic such as cookies, cakes, muffins, doughnuts, bagels, bread, pancakes, pasta, crackers, pizza, soda pop, etc. According to Dr. William Davis, the author of *Wheat Belly*, the digestion of modern-day processed wheat products yields morphine-like compounds that bind to the brain's opiate receptors, which causes a mild euphoria.[5] Milk products also produce the same good-feeling, addicting effect. So if we are feeling blue or not quite on top of things, we go directly to foods that can give us a mild high without even being aware of it. That is why they are called comfort foods. Yes, these kinds of foods actually alter our moods. They are potent enough to keep us addicted to them and so keep us on the road to an unhealthy lifestyle. Do not under estimate their powerful addictive capacities.

We often feel we are alone and that no one else has any of the problems we struggle with. However, you would be surprised how much we resemble one another and that many of us struggle with the same things to a greater or lesser degree. Most of us have battled with self-esteem issues some time or another in our lives.

> WHEN WE ARE UPSET WE TEND TO GO TO FOODS THAT GIVE US A MILD HIGH THAT WE ARE NOT EVEN AWARE OF

RECAP ON DEGENERATIVE DISEASES

Remember, in general, degenerative diseases are caused by 5 major factors:

1. Our poor-quality, nutrient deficient food choices
2. An accumulated exposure to toxins
3. Stress and negative emotions
4. Our sedentary lifestyles
5. Our unconscious negative belief system

GET HELP

Do not hesitate to ask for help. Simply opening up and talking to someone about what you are going through makes it less dramatic and more manageable. The assistance of a counsellor or another qualified person to help you visit some of your unconscious beliefs can be very beneficial.

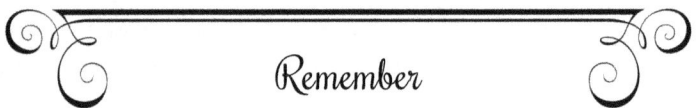

Remember

There is nothing like having a good friend or family member, someone who loves you and cares for you, to confide in. Cherish and invest in your friendships.

I believe that by having a spiritual connection with our Creator and letting His truth shine on our false beliefs, we can experience freedom from our confining low self-esteem. This relationship with God can help us dismantle these toxic, negative, limiting, deep-rooted beliefs and reprogram them to be positive, thereby affirming the person we really are. I have also listed some references to different programs that can assist you in transforming your unconscious beliefs in the Resources section at the end of the book.

SUMMARY

- **Our bodies pay the price of our longstanding bad habits.** Over the years we may develop a lot of seemingly inoffensive habits regarding our health. These bad habits accumulate with time, contributing to less than optimal health. We haven't necessarily realized that there can be any serious consequence or connection between things like regularly eating a lot of sweets or eating a heavy meal at night just before retiring for bed, and the state of our health. By taking responsibility we can retrain our habits and negative lifestyle choices. Being proactive with our health may take some determination and discipline. Do it for the love of your "buddy" – your body. You are worth it!

- **You must take responsibility by taking charge of your own personal health.** It's when you don't take action – especially when you are subject to the same societal influences as your unaware friends and family and are partaking in the same unhealthy food and lifestyle choices as they—that sooner or later you could be battling their same health issues.

- **Physical activity is an important factor to having great health and a resilient body.** Choose exercises or physical activities that you enjoy. Developing a lifelong physical exercise program helps keep our body detoxed, toned and energized. The older we get the more we have to ensure we keep moving – it's a very important key to longevity. Starting at a young age is crucial for the developing body and also lays the foundation for an important lifelong habit.

- **Realize the impact of addictions.** Despite their good intentions, it's the emotional attachment and physical addiction to certain unhealthy foods that often times prevents people from making the healthy changes they desire. Now that you know about the addictive side of comfort foods and the destruction it brings to your body, you can choose to not let this harm you any longer. Knowledge and understanding gives you the power to change things. Keep learning and get the support you need in order to apply what you learn.

- **Addressing and changing our unconscious beliefs of ourselves, or our negative self-esteem, is crucial.** Being mindful of this is important, especially if you have been experiencing repeated defeats in your efforts to make healthy changes. Know that such changes are within your reach.

Now that you have gained greater understanding of some of the root causes that have led to your illnesses, let's move on to learn what you can do to better your health.

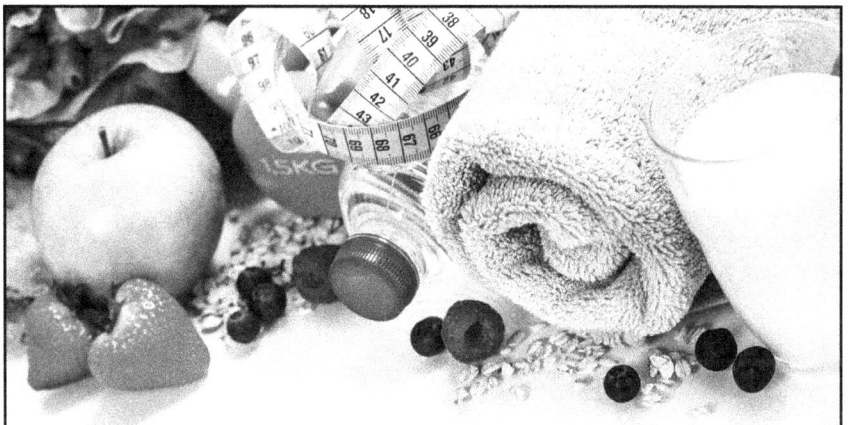

PART TWO

A Healthier You

You don't have to live in fear that the next person to come down with cancer or diabetes will be you. You can do something, whether red warning signals on your dashboard are screaming at you, or they are just starting to flicker or even if you have no signs of illness at all. The 12 Principles listed in the following chapter is an ideal place for you to start. These principles will help lay a good foundation on which you can rely to begin to rebuild a healthier you. The additional action steps listed in the last chapter will assist you and equip you to take charge of and solidify your health, giving you greater strength, energy and vitality, allowing you to live your best life ever.

Perhaps the most important decision you must make if you want to embark on this journey of getting and keeping great health is to take the first step forward: believing that you are worth it.

6

CHAPTER SIX

12 principles to guide you back to great health

From Part 1, we understand that there's a lot that we can do, and have been doing, to damage our body. However, the ways in which we can love and restore our body back to health are fairly simple and are outlined in the following 12 Principles. Let's go over these fundamental principles to help you understand what it takes to obtain the healthy, vibrant, revitalized body you were destined to have.

The 12 Principles

PRINCIPLE #1

YOU MUST EAT FOODS THAT THE HUMAN BODY WAS CREATED TO DIGEST AND ASSIMILATE.

This means we must eat whole foods, not pre-packaged foods, processed foods, fast foods or junk foods. Most of these kinds of food products contain refined carbohydrates (think white bread, pizza dough, pasta and white rice), the wrong kinds of fats and added noxious invisible substances. When broken down through the digestive process, inconsiderate of all the toxic substances the body will have to deal with, this becomes a kind of goo that sticks to our intestinal track. The texture could be compared to that of peanut butter. These sticky feces can actually stay in our body for years. With time, these residues dehydrate and become encrusted in our intestines, impairing the digestive and assimilation process. A colon detox using special herbs and fibre are needed to flush out this mucoid plaque.

It's impossible to have proper evacuation of our stools without the aid of strong fibre from raw vegetables and fruits, as well as whole grains, legumes and nuts. Fibre-rich foods act as a broom to sweep out debris, helping them not to accumulate.

Overconsumption of meat and other proteins also creates an imbalance in our digestive track. Animal proteins don't have fibre and so get reduced to a similar type of goo. We human beings are omnivores: we can eat both plant and animal foods. Not all people do, however. Some are strict vegetarians, eating only a plant-food diet. Human bodies are able to digest meat, but moderation is the key.

Meat-eating animals, in general, have shorter gastrointestinal tracts than herbivores. Carnivores are equipped with a short digestive tract, which permits the rapid evacuation of their feces. This prevents the putrefaction of the protein that causes proliferation of bacteria inside their bodies, which could lead to disease. If we consider herbivorous animals, like cows, their gastrointestinal tract is longer and more complex. Cows eat fibrous plants, which take a long time to break down. They are therefore equipped with an adapted digestive tract including several stomachs. The human body also has a longer intestinal tract than that of carnivores, although not as complex as that of a cow's. Our longer digestive tract allows us to absorb nutrients from plant foods. However, the human digestive system is also designed to allow the consumption of meat. Problems from eating meat arise when we eat it too often and in out-of-proportion quantities. One normal portion of meat is equal to the size of the palm of your hand. It is recommended to eat meat in combination with vegetables. Raw vegetables are important, as they not only supply vital phytonutrients,* but also provide the necessary fibre to ensure that the meat does not linger in the body too long causing putrefaction which leads to disease. In addition, consuming vegetables along with meat seems to aid in reducing acid reflux.

---

*plant chemicals that have been scientifically proven to provide health benefits

Furthermore, we don't necessarily need to eat meat every day, as protein is also found in other types of food such as legumes, whole grains, nuts and even vegetables. Eating one portion of meat every two days is sufficient. If you are ill, reducing the amount even more can be beneficial. If you are battling a degenerative disease like cancer, total abstinence helps to re-create an alkaline environment where cancer cells cannot thrive. Reducing the amount of meat in your diet, especially processed meats, is highly recommended in all cases. There are exceptional cases, of course, like if you are recuperating from an operation. You want to make sure you are getting sufficient good quality protein to rebuild your tissues.

If a large portion of your daily food intake does not come from healthy, whole foods that come from nature, then you will be filling up on a lot of refined products (see the following chart under Principle #2 entitled: "Unhealthy Low Glycemic Foods"). Your body does not receive proper nutrition from these highly processed foods. In addition, over the years your body can get weighed down with all those extra molecules of foreign toxic material.

Tips for Principle #1

1. Reduce intake of processed foods, fast foods and junk foods.
2. Start including more fresh whole foods in your diet. Eat a large salad, which should include a variety of vegetables, with every meal.
3. Eat less meat, particularly processed and low-quality meats.

PRINCIPLE #2

EAT FOODS IN THE RIGHT BALANCE
SO AS NOT TO SPIKE YOUR BLOOD SUGAR.

Every food has a glycemic index. Glycemic index is a measurement of the amount of glucose (sugar) released in your blood stream after digestion of a food item. The glucose in your blood has to stay within a certain narrow range. Standard fasting blood glucose readings (no food for 8 hours) are between 70-99 mg/dL (3.9-5.55 mmol/L). Commonly accepted readings after two hours are below 140 mg/dL (7.77 mmol/L).

Functional Medicine practitioners want their patient's fasting blood glucose to be under 90mg/dl (under 5 mmol/L) as anything above this is considered to be an indicator of a pre-diabetic state.

If you don't have enough glucose in your blood, you can experience dizziness, confusion and fainting. If, on the other hand, you have too much, your body goes into an alert mode. In this state, stress hormones are released, triggering the flight-or-fight survival response as well as the production of extra insulin to get rid of the over-abundant sugar that has just been released into the blood stream. When in excessive amounts, insulin is a hormone that encourages the storage of fat. Therefore an increase in insulin production leads to weight gain. These stress hormones also instruct the sympathetic nervous system to become activated. Pupils dilate to help see better, breathing is accelerated, blood pressure goes up, blood is directed to our arms and legs to supply us with extra energy to help us for fight or flight. However, the activation of the sympathetic nervous system greatly diminishes the functions of the parasympathetic system, which controls the digestive system as well as the reproductive system. This activation of stress-related hormones considerably diminishes all the rest and recovery functions of our body.

Consuming processed foods with a high glycemic index raises our blood glucose too high and subsequently lowers it too low, causing weight problems which can lead to the onset of diabetes. This, in turn, gives rise to circulation, renal and kidney dysfunction, premature aging of the arteries, as well as other kinds of degenerative diseases.

Listed below are some examples of high versus low glycemic foods. Note that most processed foods are high glycemic foods, which are detrimental to good health.

UNHEALTHY HIGH-GLYCEMIC FOODS	HEALTHY LOW-GLYCEMIC FOODS
PROCESSED CARBOHYDRATES	NATURAL WHOLE FOODS
• Cookies	• Kale
• Cakes	• Bok Choy
• Pancakes	• Spinach
• Waffles	• Romaine lettuce
• Donuts	• Cabbage
• Bread	• Green beans
• Bagels	• Tomatoes
• Muffins	• Oranges
• Crackers	• Apples
• Pasta (all pastas)	• Squash
• Pretzels	• Raw seeds
• Packaged breakfast cereals	• Nuts
• Croissants	• Legumes
• Quick-cooking oatmeal	• Avocados

If you are eating processed carbohydrates, beware: you are spiking your blood sugar! You need to eat your macronutrients, but make sure they are healthy carbohydrates, healthy proteins and healthy fats. When transitioning towards healthier eating, while still occasionally indulging in certain processed carbs, make sure that you combine them with the other types of macronutrients – such as proteins, fats and fibre – to use as a buffer so as not to spike your blood sugar.

Fats and proteins take longer to digest. If you eat them at the same time you eat a carbohydrate, it will help the glucose from the digested carbohydrate to enter the blood stream more slowly. For example, if you eat some crackers (a processed carbohydrate), make sure you eat a protein or fat at the same time.[1] Perhaps put some almond butter on your cracker. If you eat a piece of cake on some special occasion, make sure that you eat some nuts at the same time to avoid raising your blood sugar.

Tips for Principle #2

1. Eat plenty of healthy carbohydrates such as fruits and vegetables, but mostly vegetables.
2. Grains should be eaten in moderation and limited to whole grains. Millet and quinoa are excellent choices. Wild rice and brown rice are also beneficial.
3. Avoid consumption of refined carbohydrates such as pasta and bread so as to not spike your blood sugar levels.

PRINCIPLE #3

EAT NUTRIENT-DENSE FOODS.

Some foods have a higher density of minerals, vitamins, phytonutrients, enzymes and antioxidants than others. These healthy foods are even better eaten raw. When you cook your food, most of the enzymes are destroyed. Without enzymes there is no digestion. Your body does produce enzymes, but as you grow older, your reserve is continually being depleted. Include raw food with all of your meals because they contain live enzymes, which aids in digestion and can keep you from using up your own.

Listed below are some examples of good nutrient-dense foods.

- **Berries:** They are loaded with antioxidants and other phytonutrients.
  - Blueberries
  - Strawberries
  - Raspberries
  - Blackberries

- **Dark green, leafy vegetables:** Bitter plants are great for your liver; it would serve you well to eat them regularly. The more bitter vegetables can be lightly steamed to make them more edible, or you can put them in a salad or a smoothie to mask the taste and still get the benefits of eating them raw.
  - Kale
  - Dandelion greens
  - Collards
  - Watercress
  - Swiss chard
  - Spinach
  - Mustard greens
  - Arugula
  - Beet tops
  - Parsley

- **Seaweed:** This is a much-needed ingredient in our diets. It is filled with minerals as well as iodine. We are terribly deficient in iodine. Studies have shown that iodine can help prevent breast cancer and aid in detoxification, and lack of it may be the root cause of thyroid problems.[2] Please verify your source, ensuring it to be free from harmful contaminants.

Fats and proteins are also beneficial nutrient-dense foods.

- **Good healthy fats:** Add lots of good healthy fats such as cold pressed virgin olive oil, non-refined coconut oil, even fats from good-quality, grass-fed meats and butter to your diet. The 0% fat fad is out! Fats are good for us; we are in desperate need of them.

- **Vegetable oils:** Salad and cooking oils, like hydrogenated or refined soybean oil and corn oil, are widely used in the snack food and processed food industry. Hydrogenated oils are trans fats and therefore harmful. They also cause inflammation because they contain pro-inflammatory omega-6 fatty acids. They are also GMO oils coming from "Roundup Ready" crops. The herbicide Roundup® contains a toxic active ingredient called *glyphosate* which destroys good gut bacteria and impedes nutrient absorption. Canola oil is also a GMO oil and so should equally be avoided. We must take precautionary measure to eliminate or drastically reduce the intake of these refined vegetable oils in our diet.

Using small amounts of unrefined, expeller or cold pressed oils such as sunflower, safflower, sesame or grape seed is beneficial.

- **Omega-3 fish oil supplements:** These oils protect against inflammation and heart disease. Omega-3 fish oils are extracted from cold-water fish such as salmon, mackerel, sardines and anchovies. Make sure that your source is free of heavy metals and pesticides.

Other great sources of Omega-3 oils are:
- Chia seeds
- Walnuts
- Flaxseeds

- **Raw nuts and seeds:** They are an excellent source of good-quality protein as well as a good source of healthy fats. Their nutritional value is increased when soaked or sprouted.
- **Good quality animal protein:** Meat and organ meat coming from grass fed animals, non-polluted fish, as well as pasture-raised chickens, although more expensive than what we find in our traditional grocery stores, are all good options. Pasture-raised chicken eggs are also an excellent nutrient-dense food.

Tips for Principle #3

1. Include a large spectrum of vibrant colours in your daily plant food choices, such as berries and dark green, leafy vegetables; all loaded with antioxidants and phytonutrients.

2. Remember to take your anti-inflammatory omega-3 oils and to include a lot of good quality fats in your diet. Eliminate your usage of refined vegetable oils containing inflammatory omega-6 fatty acids.

3. Add small portions of good-quality animal protein as well as raw nuts and seeds (soaked or sprouted would even be better).

PRINCIPLE #4

CONSUME MORE FIBRE AND ADD PROBIOTICS TO YOUR DIET.

There are two types of fibre: soluble and insoluble. We need both in our diet. Soluble fibre is fibre that dissolves or swells when put into water. Soluble fibres bind with fatty acids and slow digestion, enabling sugars to be released more slowly into the body, thereby helping to regulate blood sugar levels. These fibres also help lower LDL and VLDL, the "bad" cholesterol. Beans, fruits, flaxseed, oats and oat bran are especially good sources of soluble fibre.

Certain types of soluble fibre can also function as a prebiotic. Inulin and other prebiotic fibre, as well as resistant starch, are good food ingredients that nourish the beneficial bacteria (probiotic) necessary for the maintaining of a healthy gut flora. Chicory root, Jerusalem artichoke, dandelion greens, garlic, leeks, onions, asparagus, apples, wheat bran, oats, flax seeds, yacon root (yellow sweet potato), konjac root, burdock root, cocoa, banana and jicama–besides being good sources of fibre–contain either prebiotic fibre or resistant starch.

Insoluble fibre does not dissolve in water. It helps hydrate and move waste through the intestines. Insoluble fibre increases stool volume, and retains water in the colon thus helping to provide a larger, softer stool. This type of fibre is therefore great for preventing constipation. All plants, especially vegetables, whole grains and brown rice are full of insoluble fibre.

The Mayo Clinic gives the following daily recommendations of fibre for adults.[3]

GENDER	AGE 50 OR YOUNGER	AGE 51 OR OLDER
MEN	38 grams	30 grams
WOMEN	25 grams	21 grams

This recommendation is a good place to start, as most of us don't even reach this minimum. In pre-industrialized societies daily fibre intake was 50 and sometimes even up to 100 grams per day. Although we probably won't be consuming 100 grams of fibre per day, just know that it would be beneficial to consume more than the minimal recommendation.

It's important to get fibre from whole foods because these contain many other healthful plant compounds such as antioxidants, and many important phytonutrients. Dietary fibres are found naturally not only in fruits and vegetables, but also in legumes, nuts and whole grains. A medium-sized apple contains about 4 grams of fibre. If your daily fibre intake from whole foods is not sufficient, supplementing your diet with a multi-fibre blend is a great place to start to get immediate health benefits.

Probiotics and fermented foods:

Adding in a good-quality probiotic supplement is very important for gut health. Fermented foods are also an excellent source of probiotics. Fermented vegetables such as sauerkraut or kimchi, or even fermented dairy such as kefir or homemade yoghurt made from organic, grass-fed cow's milk, have a wide range of health benefits. You will most definitely want to resort to fermented foods or a probiotic supplement if ever you have to take antibiotics, thus enabling your intestinal flora to recover.

Fermented foods or supplemental probiotics also strengthen your immune system, reduce urinary tract infections, and help with constipation or diarrhoea. They also help improve inflammatory bowel conditions, including leaky gut. Leaky gut is a term used when one has an increased intestinal permeability. This allows partially digested food and toxins to pass into the blood stream, causing food sensitivities, thyroid as well as autoimmune conditions. Probiotics may also help ease the discomforts of premenstrual syndrome and improve mood by releasing more of the neurotransmitter serotonin. They also augment the nutritional content of food, and may even help you absorb many more nutrients from the foods you eat. Introducing fermented foods as well as prebiotic fibre into your daily diet may be one of the most important things you can you do for the improvement of your health.

Make sure that these fermented foods are raw, naturally fermented and that they do not contain white vinegar. Pickled vegetables using white vinegar do not have the same health properties as naturally fermented foods. While distilled white vinegar is not something I choose to keep in my kitchen pantry, as it lacks the probiotic properties of "live", unpasteurized vinegars such as found in apple cider vinegar, it is very useful as a natural, nontoxic household cleaner.

Tips for Principle #4

1. Keep increasing your vegetable consumption in order to increase your fibre intake, making sure to include vegetables that also contain prebiotic fibre or resistant starch.

2. Gradually start adding in fermented foods to ensure excellent gut health.

and/or

3. Add a fibre mixture (which also contains some prebiotic fibre) to your soups or smoothies daily.

4. Include a reputable probiotic supplement.

PRINCIPLE #5

KEEP YOUR ACID-BASE BALANCE STABLE.

All foods have a certain acidic or alkaline measurement. Eating too many highly acidic foods disturbs the optimum functioning of the body. High levels of acidity will actually start to corrode your body tissue, causing inflammation inside your body. If left unchecked, this acidity will disturb the smooth functioning of your organism. You are made up of trillions of cells, and if they are not functioning properly, your health will be compromised. Acidified body cells become weak and lead to unhealthy body tissue. Chronic acidity and inflammation is a major root cause of sickness and disease. Cancer cannot be present in an alkaline environment, but it thrives in an acidic environment. This is why it is so important to make sure you eat sufficient amounts of alkaline foods.

Start decreasing the amount of acid-forming foods you eat, and start increasing alkaline-forming foods. For optimum health, your diet should be comprised of 80% alkaline-forming foods and 20% acidic-based foods. Consumption of large quantities of acidic foods, especially meat, processed carbohydrates, sugar and particularly added fructose, puts an enormous strain on the kidneys. Consuming alkaline foods can quickly relieve acidic build-up. In an alkaline environment, your body will begin to regain its health.

Remember

As a general rule, all protein and most grains and nuts are acidifying. All raw vegetables and fruits are alkalizing.

Here is a general list of acidic- and alkaline-forming foods. The list is based on the PRAL index, which stands for Potential Renal Acid Load, originally developed to measure the acid-base level of food.[4] It has since been widely used to help identify potentially kidney-damaging foods.

ACIDIC FOODS	**ALKALINE FOODS**
• Red meats	• Parsley
• Pork	• Celery
• Poultry	• Radishes
• Fish	• Tomatoes
• Eggs	• Leeks
• Dairy	• Apples
• Wheat (and most other grains)	• Apricots
• Beans	• Bananas
• Nuts	• Cherries
• Fruit beverages	• Raw Seeds

It's so important to always include some kind of raw vegetable at each of your meals to ensure a sufficient supply of minerals to counteract the acidity of the proteins and other cooked foods of the meal. Leafy vegetables are loaded with necessary minerals, including calcium, to keep your body in the correct pH balance. The healthier you want to be, the more energy and vitality you want to have, the more you need to include all kinds of raw, green leafy vegetables in your diet. They are by far the highest alkaline contributor. Just remember that once the vegetables are cooked, their alkalizing capacity decreases.

Although it might seem contradictory, citrus fruits actually have an alkalinizing effect in the body. These acidic fruits, once digested, create an alkaline ash. A great way to start the day is to press half a lemon or lime in a large glass of pure water to help de-acidify and detoxify your body.

Tips for Principle #5

1. Make sure that at least half of your plate is filled with raw and cooked vegetables; the rest can be whole grains or proteins. Work up to 60/40. For superb health, or for a detoxifying diet, work up to 80/20.

PRINCIPLE #6

DRINK SUFFICIENT AMOUNTS OF WATER.

Your body is composed of approximately 60% water. Fluid from your body is continuously lost through skin evaporation, breathing, urine and stools. A typical adult can lose as much as two to three quarts (about two to three litres) daily. You must replace the water you lose to prevent dehydration and to ensure optimal bodily functions. The usual recommendation is eight 8-ounce glasses per day, which is equivalent to about 2 litres, or half a gallon. A formula you can use to estimate your particular recommended daily water intake in ounces is to calculate a ½ ounce of water for each pound of body weight. For example if you weighed 130 lbs., you would calculate half of that amount in ounces. Example: 130 x ½ which would equal 65 oz. divided by 8 oz. = 8.1 cups of water or 2 litres. This is one formula; there are others you can use. Depending on your particular situation, there are several other factors to take into consideration – such as your level of physical activity or the climate – in order to assess the precise amount your body requires at any given time.

Drinking pure, clean water is essential for good health. Tap water contains chemicals, notably chlorine, and in most cities fluoride, which are both toxic to our body. You can purchase large water containers in most local grocery stores. Many grocery stores also provide a water distribution machine that filters water through various procedures, allowing you to refill your bottle with safe, clean water for an effective quality/price option.

Children who are not encouraged and guided to drink water early in their lives will become dependent on soft drinks and juices, setting them up for dehydration, says Dr. F Batmanghelidj, author of *Your Body's Many Cries for Water*. He also considers chronic dehydration as a disease producer. He states: "It is chronic water shortage in the body that causes most of the diseases of the human body."[5]

Many people don't realize the importance of simply drinking water. It's not the same as drinking other liquids. Here are several reasons why your body needs water:

- Water is a solvent. It dissolves nutrients so that they can pass through the intestinal cell walls into your bloodstream. It also carries these nutrients through your veins to be distributed to every cell and organ in your body. It also carries away toxins through the lymph.
- Water helps maintain normal bowel function. Adequate water intake allows the proper movement of your stools through the gastrointestinal tract, which prevents constipation.
- Water helps your kidneys carry waste products out of your body. Your kidneys cleanse and rid your body of toxins. Consume adequate intake of fluids in order to support this process. Chronically drinking too little water makes you prone to kidney stones.
- Your cells need to be plump to be able to do their job effectively. If they lack water, they shrivel up and normal function is severely restrained.
- Water helps keep your skin moist. Dehydration makes your skin dry and prone to wrinkles. Dry skin can be improved with proper hydration.
- Water is a conductor for the electrical messages sent between cells. This supports and permits many bodily functions, such as enabling your many muscles to move, your eyes to see and even the brain to process.
- Your body temperature is regulated with water. This is done by cooling and through perspiration.
- Weight control is much easier when you drink lots of water. We often eat when in fact we are simply thirsty.

You must have water in your diet; it helps you to be well nourished. You can't live without it. Coffee, tea and soft drinks do not have the same function as water. These types of beverages can actually dehydrate your body and add to the digestive load. To aid with digestion and even with weight loss, drink 20 minutes before a meal and not until two hours after eating so as to not dilute your digestive enzymes.

Tips for Principle #6

1. Take a bottle of water (preferably glass or stainless steel) with you everywhere you go, and drink away!

PRINCIPLE #7

INCREASE YOUR VITAMINS, MINERALS, ANTIOXIDANTS AND PHYTONUTRIENTS THROUGH SUPPLEMENTATION.

Vitamin and mineral supplements are intended to enrich your diet, not take the place of real food or healthy meals. They can't replace all of the nutrients and benefits of consuming whole foods. Food contains thousands of phytochemicals, fibre and other vitamins and minerals that work together to promote good health. Whole foods must therefore occupy a central place in your diet. However, the nutritional quality of fruits and vegetables in today's farming practices is compromised and doesn't contain the amounts of nutrients needed for optimal health. Many trace minerals, enzymes, antioxidants and vitamins are not available in high enough quantities in the food we purchase from the grocery stores today. Besides, we aren't eating enough of them to begin with. Taking high-quality supplements is simply unavoidable. We need to provide our body with optimal amounts of vitamins, minerals, micronutrients, trace elements and antioxidants in a balanced and bioavailable form in order for it to function optimally.

The Centers for Disease Control and Prevention have reported the following:

In 2013, 13.1% of [American adults] met fruit intake recommendations, (…) and 8.9% met vegetable recommendations.[6]

Data from the National Health and Nutrition Examination Survey (NHANES) indicate that:[7]

- 93% of Americans don't get enough vitamin E
- 56% don't get enough magnesium
- 44% don't get enough vitamin A
- 31% don't get enough vitamin C
- 14% don't get enough vitamin B6
- 12% don't get enough zinc
- Many lack vitamin D.

The Journal of American Medical Association (JAMA) confirms that there are known health benefits to taking supplements.[8] They are helpful when it comes to providing the missing nutrients in your diet. But don't trust just any product simply because it's in the health food store. Quality varies greatly from one product to another. Many supplements are inadequate, and some are even detrimental to your health. Some are well known because of the advertisements that make them so, but in reality, they produce few health benefits. Do your research, and find a good-quality supplement that comes in a balanced and bioavailable form.[9] Then remember to take them every day. They won't do you any good if you forget to take them.

Tips for Principle #7

1. Take good quality supplements every day. Set up a routine of taking them with meals.

PRINCIPLE #8

GET SUFFICIENT EXERCISE AND ADEQUATE SUNSHINE.

Your body was made to be mobile. In our modern society, it's too easy to go through the day barely even moving. We get in the car, park the closest to the entrance, take the elevator to our work space, work for hours in front of a computer screen, and then come home and rest in front of the TV! We are thus obliged to find reasons to move.

Taking fitness classes or imposing on ourselves a brisk, daily walk may seem a superfluous activity; it is not! Regular physical activity is necessary for staying healthy and staving off disease. The movement of lymph depends on the movement of our muscles. Lymph carries away and neutralizes harmful bacteria and other debris so that the blood doesn't get overloaded. As explained in chapter 3, our lymphatic system (our internal waste treatment system) does not have a heart muscle to push the fluids along, the way our blood vessels have. Everything gets backed up when our lymph doesn't move. We become lethargic and prone to disease.

Vigorous exercise not only helps move our lymph, but also helps us sweat, which helps remove toxins through our skin. Be prudent, as one can experience drawbacks from over-exercising. If you are chronically overly stressed, your adrenals are suffering; participating in intense workouts continues to exhaust your adrenals making you even more tired. It's important to wash or shower after an intense workout so that your body doesn't reabsorb these toxins. Try to have a good sweat at least once a week – three times is even better. If you can't bring your body to eliminate toxins through perspiration by exercising, then taking a sauna is a good alternative; an infrared sauna is even better for deep removal of toxins. It also aids to combat stress as it helps with relaxation. Remember to drink plenty of water to replace the fluids you will be losing and be sure to include healthy supplements to keep important electrolytes in balance.

Moving your body more vigorously also helps it take in more oxygen; this also helps with the removal of toxins through the lungs. Try doing your exercises outdoors to take advantage of the fresh air and to take in much needed sunshine, which helps expose us to doses of critically needed vitamin D.

Tips for Principle #8

1. Start some kind of exercise program, even if it is only brisk walking for 15 to 30 minutes three times per week. Work up to 30 minutes daily.

2. Get outdoors as much as you can. Expose yourself to adequate amounts of safe sunshine to help build up your critically needed vitamin D supply.

3. Take an adequate, good quality vitamin D supplement, especially if you live in the Nordic regions and especially during the winter months where exposure to sunshine is limited.

PRINCIPLE #9

GET YOUR BEAUTY SLEEP

Emerging science and advances in technology have permitted researchers to examine how adequate sleep, or lack of it, positively or negatively affects our health. Sleep scientists are now able to state that an adequate amount of sleep provides more benefits than previously thought. According to the National Sleep Foundation, adults need from seven to nine hours of sleep daily for optimum health. Studies have shown a growing link between inadequate sleep and serious health problems, including diabetes, high blood pressure, memory loss and depression. Sleep loss also appears to stimulate appetite, which can contribute to obesity.[10]

One short-term study conducted by the National Sleep Foundation found a correlation between inadequate sleep and insufficient levels of the hormone leptin, the hormone responsible for the feeling of satiety. Adequate levels of leptin signal satiety to the brain and suppresses appetite. Low levels of leptin causes the body to crave high fat and high-carbohydrate foods. Sleep deprivation can also lead to diabetes by impairing sugar metabolism and decreasing the capacity to process blood glucose, which increases the production of insulin.[11]

When you're resting, your body is no longer in action mode and does not need to pump as much blood, so your blood pressure and heart rate decrease. Blood pressure slows down at night so your cardiac muscle and circulatory system have time to relax and repair. Over the course of 20 years, researchers in Britain have observed how sleep patterns affected civil servants' mortality rate. They found that people who got five to seven hours of sleep or less a night were almost twice as likely to die from all causes. Lack of sleep especially increased one's risk of death from cardiovascular issues nearly two-fold![12]

I'm sure you have all heard the saying, "Go to bed early so that you can get your beauty sleep." Well, there actually is some truth to that. When you don't get enough sleep, your body releases more cortisol, the stress hormone. In excess amounts, cortisol can break down skin collagen, the protein that keeps your skin from wrinkling, and can leave you with fine lines and old-looking skin. You can also get puffy eyes when you haven't had a good night's sleep. And when lack of sleep is chronic, you can get dark circles under your eyes.

Furthermore, your body is regulated by a 24-hour circadian rhythm. This acts like an internal clock and is regulated by sunlight and darkness. When the sun starts to go down, your internal clock signals your body to slowly start changing its activities. When night falls, your body is primed for rest and restoration as well as the detoxification of all of your body parts. If you don't get to bed on time, your body won't be regenerated sufficiently. Sleep is essential to help maintain mood, memory and the ability to concentrate. It plays a key role in the proper functioning of your endocrine (hormonal) system as well as your immune system.

When we think of sleep, we think of shutting down and resting. However, even though metabolism slows down, other important processes, many still unknown to scientists, are taking place. Sleep allows your body to rest, repair and rebuild from the wear and tear of the day.

Tips for Principle #9

1. Go to bed before 11 pm, 10 pm is ideal and try to get seven to eight hours of good sleep.

PRINCIPLE #10

REDUCE YOUR EXPOSURE TO TOXINS

You are surrounded by all kinds of toxins. Often the greatest exposure to toxins is found in your own home. From kitchen cleaners, non-stick cookware and plastic storage containers in the kitchen, to cleaning and disinfectant products and aerosol sprays to mask odours in the bathroom, as well as preservatives in your personal care products, you are being bombarded. Be aware of what you are exposing yourself to.

It may be impossible to cut all toxins out of your home, but you can start to reduce the amount you are exposed to. One place to start is by verifying the personal care products and perfumes that you put directly on your skin. You can begin to eliminate skin care products that contain one family of toxic preservatives called parabens (methyl, propyl, butyl and ethyl). These bacteria killing preservatives are also cytotoxic, which means that they are toxic to our cells; when we put these creams on our bodies they cause cellular damage.[13] For this reason, doctors warn not to use adult skin care products on your baby's skin. Remember that hand sanitizers may also contain parabens. Be careful when it comes to using them on your children.

Formaldehyde, a cancer-causing chemical, is used as a preservative in cosmetics because it is also highly effective at killing microbes.[14] Cosmetic, clothing and furniture manufacturers use formaldehyde-release-agents in order to release small amounts of this chemical a little at a time, thereby prolonging protection from bacterial proliferation in their products. These can be listed on labels as:

- Quaternium 15
- 2-bromo-2-nitroprorane-1,3 diol
- Diazolidinyl urea
- DMDM hydantoin

If you use facial creams that contain preservatives, and you add to that aerosol hair spray, antiperspirants containing toxic aluminum, nail polish, perfume, makeup and lipstick, the level of toxicity to which you have exposed yourself has jumped up several notches. Your seemingly innocuous morning bathroom ritual has set you up for a day of toxicity – and you haven't even stepped out the door!

Don't forget about the emotional toxins that wreak havoc in your body, especially when you harbour grudges and bitterness for extended periods of time. We talked about stress hormones, which over time eventually produce inflammation, the precursor of all disease. These hormones also shut down, or at least slow down, the parasympathetic nervous system, which is responsible for activating the rest and repair cycle. Digestion and assimilation, as well as reproductive function and fertility, are also impaired. Toxic emotions destabilize us in many ways. Release these emotions from your body by communicating with someone who can help you resolve the hurt or disappointment you are hanging on to. Writing about your thoughts and feelings in a journal is also helpful. This provides a safe environment that helps initiate the forgiving process.

Tips for Principle #10

1. Start small; reduce one or two toxic contaminants in your home. For example: do away with one preservative-containing product that you put directly on your skin, such as a moisturizer or a night cream, and replace it with a more natural preservative-free cream.
2. Take some action to de-stress your life. Put in place some healthy boundaries in your personal and work life. Reduce your workload if necessary.
3. Cleanse yourself of toxic emotions by beginning the process of forgiveness.

PRINCIPLE #11

RELAX. BE GRATEFUL

Some of us are introverts, while others are extroverts. Being extroverted means replenishing and refuelling ourselves by being around people, whereas being introverted means refuelling and gaining energy from being away from people. Regardless, everyone needs some down time to just be alone.

If we are always on the go, constantly keeping ourselves busy, we tend to burn out. We are no longer efficient in taking good care of ourselves, nor can we be sympathetic to the needs of those around us. Relaxation is a key to good health and a great stress reliever. When you take time to relax, you become more sensitive to your own needs. You are taking care of yourself because you are being respectful of your body's limits. Taking time to relax tells your body that you care about it, that it gets to just hang out and not be pressured to do anything. This allows you to take a break from those responsibilities weighing on your shoulders.

Relaxation helps trigger the parasympathetic nervous system, which activates the rest and restoration cycle your body needs to be balanced and healthy. Your body and your psyche need down time to replenish and restore. Practice deep-breathing exercises. Breathing in deeply and slowly and exhaling in the same way several times in a row is a simple way to reduce stress. This can be done at any moment, even in the middle of a stressful workday. Results can be experienced in just a matter of minutes. Deep breathing activates the parasympathetic nervous system, which not only reduces stress but also induces relaxation.

Practicing gratefulness is also a wonderful habit to get into. It trains your brain to focus on positive things. This slows you down from your habitually fast-paced way of living life and helps your brain to steer away from the negative and focus on the positive. You feel lighter, more radiant and dynamic. This practice also improves digestion, assimilation and absorption of foods.

Tips for Principle #11

1. Allow yourself some down time with no pressure to do anything in particular. You can unwind by taking a stroll in the park or by taking a relaxing bath.
2. Practice deep breathing exercises regularly, including when you are stressed.
3. Plan some time every day to be by yourself, to just relax and acknowledge the things you are grateful for. You can do this by simply sitting just ten minutes to reflect, to connect with God or to journal.

PRINCIPLE #12

ENJOY LIFE. BE FILLED WITH JOY. CONTRIBUTE.

It is extremely important to take a break from work and performance and to take time to have fun and enjoy life, especially by spending time with people who are important to us. We are not meant to be loners. Creating joyful memories with people contributes to a well-balanced life. Reminiscing over these joyful memories together continues to create joy.

Our brain, which is the control-centre for almost all of the processes of our body, functions optimally when we are in joy. It's like the lubricating oil for the cogs and gears of our brain. A joyful brain is a healthy brain, and a healthy brain produces a healthy body.

Everyone needs to feel liked, accepted, appreciated and seen. Make a habit of recognizing the good in others and let them know that you care for them. We all have some altruistic streak in us. Sooner or later in life, and to a greater or lesser degree, we all want to feel that we have contributed somehow to something that helps create a better world or helps improve the lives of others. Contributing with our gifts in some way, however insignificant it may seem, offers the potential of bringing us – and others – great joy. Life goes by way too fast. Take action now. Don't underestimate the impact of your contribution.

Tips for Principle #12

1. Do one fun activity with your family or friends once a week. If that's a stretch for you, plan something once a month. The importance of this is to do it consistently.

2. Find a way to contribute to bettering someone's life on a regular basis.

3. Smile. A smile goes a long way.

7

CHAPTER SEVEN

Getting started

In addition to the 12 Principles, included here are some practical action steps to help you get started. In order for you to be successful in developing healthier habits in your life, I want to encourage you to become more aware of what is happening in and outside of your body, and to become more attentive of your mental and emotional conditions. Be conscious of how your body is feeling in general, and be thoughtful of how your habits, thoughts and health are all interconnected in this process. Decide which of these principles you will want to start out with and at what level you can implement them. Accept and respect wherever you are as you begin your new journey.

A GLOBAL UNDERSTANDING OF YOUR BODY

As a review of what we have learned in Part 1 of this book, food and liquids do not simply go in through one end and out the other without having an impact on the rest of our body while in transit. When we eat junk food, it gets digested and goes to every cell of our body. Understanding the negative impact and insidious damage this has been doing to our body is essential: habitually eating these kinds of foods will cause damage. Fortunately, we are now no longer ignorant of these things. If you have a tendency to forget this cause and effect reality, observe all the sickness and disease so prevalent in today's ubiquitous fast- and processed-food society. Use this as a constant reminder that eating refined food does cause health problems.

What is important to grasp regarding disease, is that if one particular part of our body is sick, the remaining parts are equally at risk. It's just that one particular body part has broken down first, probably because it was genetically the weakest part. As a recap, if you look only at the obviously sick part of your body and try to treat it solely by taking medication or surgically removing it, you will never obtain total health. Even if it has been medically treated or surgically removed, the rest of your organism is still bathing in the same less-than-optimal, acidic, inflamed condition as before the intervention. It therefore remains, prone to disease. It may just be a matter of time before you come down with another illness. This breakdown will no doubt occur in the next genetically weakest part of your body. Unless of course you have been proactively dealing with the root cause and doing your part to improve your diet and lifestyle.

Please remember, every part of our body is interconnected with all the other parts. It's not because we isolate and treat a particular part of our anatomy that the rest of our body will regain its health. Let's learn to cultivate and care for our entire body in a holistic way. We must also learn to direct our attention to, and address the root causes of, our illnesses.

Taking a holistic approach not only includes making dietary changes, but also increasing your physical activity, making changes to any harmful, negative thought patterns and removing yourself from any chronically toxic and stressful environments. Surprisingly, stress reduction can often be accomplished by changing our perception of the situation. Adding in some personal self-care as well as exercise can also do wonders to combat stress.

> YOU HELP EVERY CELL IN YOUR BODY WHEN YOU NOURISH YOURSELF WITH HEALTHY WHOLE FOOD

As you begin to eat healthy whole foods, nourishment will be made available to all parts of your body, to every single cell, rebuilding your immune system and making your body stronger and more resilient. Partaking in physical exercise will oxygenate, detoxify and help you gain muscle, building a robust foundation of strength. In addition, doing things that bring you joy will bring balance and zest to your life. Finally, mustering up the courage to deal with your emotional toxicity, which is often times at the root of our ailments, will bring healing and freedom to your life.

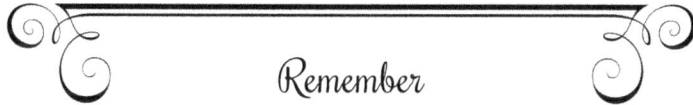

Every part of our body is interconnected with all the other parts. Your whole body needs to restore in order to really be healthy. A whole body approach is truly necessary for effective healing and optimal health.

BE AWARE OF THE SIGNALS ON YOUR DASHBOARD

Again, as a reminder, start paying attention to those little aches and pains you are experiencing. Your body (who is also actually your "buddy", remember) is gently letting you know that there is something starting to go wrong. Start analyzing when you become aware of them or when you get sick. Ask yourself:

- What was the last thing I ate, or what did I eat the day before I got sick?
- Did anything of significance happen just before I got sick?
- Was I under a lot of stress?
- Was I feeling huge amounts of rejection?
- Was I angry or furious at someone? Perhaps even unconsciously?
- In general, what kind of food have I been eating over the past days or weeks and even months? Has it been nutrient dense or void of nutrients?

You will begin to see patterns. Take note, for instance, how many people get sick just after Halloween or during the Christmas holidays when there has been an overindulgence of festive foods. The cold weather is often to blame. I challenge you to eat a sugar-free (remember, carbs are sugars) Christmas and see, even if it is cold outside or there are huge temperature changes, whether you get sick or not. You will begin to observe and see just how often you get sick right after some kind of food indulgence of sugar or other refined, high-glycemic carbohydrate. This makes sense as sugar is an immune suppressor – remember?

If you wake up in the morning with stiff joints, this could indicate that you are having problems with acidity or overall congestion of your body. Examine what you have been eating or have indulged in over the past weeks or months and even years. Red meats and HFCS (high fructose corn syrup) can cause uric acid build up in the joints. To help remove toxins, try modifying your diet, initiating a short fast, drinking more water or mobilizing your body by becoming more physically active for the next couple of days, and see if you still wake up with the same problem. Consider your emotions to see if you are angry, stressed or bitter. Bitterness can cause inflammation of the joints. Negative emotions cause stress and stress releases too much cortisol which produces inflammation. You may need to initiate forgiveness, accept your situation and exercise letting go. Practice deep breathing exercises to help you relax and de-stress. Our "dashboard" signals may seem insignificant, but on the contrary, they reveal that there is a problem that needs tending to.

Make notes in your calendar or journal, or even get a special notebook to record and track your health analysis. You may notice that sometimes several different circumstances combine to contribute to your having a weakened immune system. Perhaps there were several days in a row when you didn't get enough sleep. Possibly you were stressed out at work or because of some other conflict. Or maybe your feelings of abandonment, rejection or sadness made you want to eat more carbs to try to alter your mood so that you wouldn't feel so rotten. You will begin to notice how all of these things together weaken your body and create a terrain where microbes and illness can flourish. Be your own best detective.

I urge you, if you have warning signs on your dashboard, or are suffering from any kind of degenerative disease, please begin immediately to evaluate your situation. Then change harmful aspects of your lifestyle and modify your diet, whether you think you are eating healthily or not. Interestingly enough, most everyone thinks they eat healthily.

If you have some kind of recurring "mysterious" pain or tend to get sick regularly with a flu, sore throats, ear aches, etc., please don't live in denial, blaming a flu bug, or some other reason, but rather take responsibility. Don't put off facing what you don't want to face, it only gets worse with time. There is most definitely a root issue causing this repetitive symptom.

Catch it while it is in its beginning stages. Observe, and you will start to understand that either you are not receiving the nourishment your body needs, you've been exposed to too many toxins, or there are some unattended, underlying emotional issues, or a combination of these factors. Symptoms don't lie.

> *Most men would rather deny a hard truth than face it.*
> – George R.R. Martin

Don't be like "most men"! Value yourself and face your issues.

> *It's only after you've stepped outside your comfort zone that you begin to change, grow, and transform.*
> – Roy T. Bennett

REDUCE THE INTAKE OF WHEAT FLOUR PRODUCTS

Take note that one of the most widespread detrimental foods in our society today is processed wheat products. It is amazing to observe to what extent a huge proportion of the food we eat is made from processed wheat flour. We are eating this high-glycemic index carbohydrate at almost every meal. Toast for breakfast, sandwiches for lunch, pasta for supper, as well as muffins or cookies for snacks. We are simply eating too much of this refined grain. A simple and effective way to help restore your health is to stop eating all processed carbohydrates. Once you feel better, you can perhaps eat some wheat products again, but never to the extent that you were eating them in the past. Eating too many processed carbohydrates is very probably a big part of what got you sick in the first place. It stands to reason that if you return to eating the same things you ate before, you will get sick again.

Again, if you are experiencing any kind of illness, you can be certain that your body terrain is over acidic and inflamed. To remedy this, all the while healing your whole body and preventing new illnesses from developing, reduce the ingestion of processed and acidifying foods like bread, pasta, cookies, cakes, doughnuts, waffles, as well as other types of processed snack foods, and start eating more alkalizing whole foods.

Reducing your carbohydrate intake in this manner will invariably increase your appetite, and that hunger should be satisfied with the most alkalizing foods on the planet – vegetables. Add to this healthy, satiating fats and healthy sources of protein. These types of foods also have the benefits of having a low glycemic index. As you begin to nourish yourself with beneficial foods, you will be helping every cell in your body to perform at its best.

As previously mentioned, as we incorporate natural means to treat our illnesses we are also helping to bring restoration to our whole body. As an example, if you start drinking more water to aid with a bladder infection, the extra water will not only be available to your bladder but also to all the cells in your body. Actually, drinking adequate amounts of water may well be preventing you from contracting many other health challenges.

You may be struggling with your health and cannot seem to find a reason why. Or perhaps you are living in a situation that puts you under a lot of harmful stress and you conclude that there is nothing you can do to improve your situation. This can be discouraging and overwhelming. Chronic stress is not conducive to having an energized healthy body. To get out of that rut and change things around, perhaps you could start asking yourself some thought-provoking questions, something like: "What is the payoff of me giving up on my health?" Another question could be: "How is putting myself down or feeling sorry for myself serving me?", or "Is it possible that my perception of what is going on biased? Am I open enough to consider a different perspective?" You may find that these questions are not necessarily appropriate in all cases, but they can be a starting point. These may be radical questions, but they have the potential to bring about radical positive changes. Don't put up with mistreating your body, or letting any situation or circumstance destroy you any longer. After all, it's YOUR body and YOUR health! Loving yourself is where you need to start if you want to bring lasting results.

Every body is different, so get to know yours well. Even if you think you are eating healthy, be on guard. Don't compare yourself with what others are doing or eating, as this will get you off track. If you notice signs on your dashboard, attend to them.

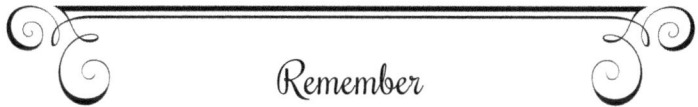

Most anyone who is not proactively taking steps to eat and live well is most likely having health problems. It just might not be so evident in that moment.

To reiterate, please don't let yourself go astray by comparing; just listen and really tune in to the signs your body is emitting. Signs may be in the form of headaches, constipation, skin rashes, abdominal pain, sleepiness, exhaustion, insomnia or the like. Use these signs as evidence from your "buddy", who is trying to help you become aware of some repetitive actions that are doing you harm.

PROFESSIONAL "DASHBOARD LIGHT" DETECTORS

Your dashboard lights – your symptoms – are early warning signs that may help you detect problems even before they show up on medical exams. Stop, analyze and then decide to change something to improve your health. Even taking a small step gets you heading in the right direction. And if you act immediately, you have an excellent chance of reversing the early stages of an illness before it can do you further harm. Your body is amazing. It wants to heal. But it needs your help. If you don't know how to read your symptoms (the signs on your dashboard), get help from alternative health care professionals.

To get to the bottom of degenerative diseases, you need to address the root issues. Listen to your body and learn how it works. Know that healthy foods and healthy lifestyle changes are needed in order to have true health. There is no other way.

Eating healthy, whole foods will help your whole body get healthy.

This is practicing preventive medicine. In doing so, you will be applying Hippocrates's counsel: "Let food be thy medicine and medicine be thy food". If you find this too much of a challenge to do by yourself, try consulting an alternative health practitioner. Listen to what this person has to say. Try out what is proposed to you and you will surely benefit from the results.

Following is a list of some professional "dashboard-light detectors":
- Iridologists
- Reflexologists
- Live blood and dry blood analysis technicians
- Osteopaths
- Acupuncturists

Others who can help you get started on the right nutritional foods, or herbs that your body needs to repair itself are:
- Naturopaths
- Herbalists
- Certified health coaches
- Bio-nutritionists
- Nutrition coaches
- Functional Medicine practitioners

NINE ACTION STEPS

As you begin to make the proposed changes to your diet and lifestyle, your body will begin to restore from the inside out. In time you will feel so much better and have more energy. You might start by making only small, incremental changes, and sometimes you will fall back. Don't get discouraged. Just get back up and keep going. Every small step that you take will make a difference in the long run. It doesn't matter how long it takes to master a new healthy habit, feel empowered because you are heading in the right direction by starting.

- **Step 1: Begin experimenting with the 12 Principles.** Applying all of these principles may take time, practice and determination. New actions won't become engrained habits overnight. Look over all 12 principles, and pat yourself on the back for the ones that you are implementing, no matter to what degree. For those that you have not yet implemented, decide which ones you want to start with. Start small and focus on consistency. It's amazing how a little effort can go a long way. Be encouraged; every little bit adds up. Taking care of your body does require an investment, but it will be so worth it. If you start and fail, don't worry; that's par for the course, just get back up and keep going. Get together with a friend or a group of friends and do this together. This not only makes the process more pleasant, but also helps to keep you accountable and motivated.

- **Step 2: Start analyzing the nutrient content of the foods you eat.** Remember our cells need a lot of micronutrients to function optimally. Start being aware of how many processed foods you actually eat, and perhaps how few whole foods you eat. Track how many garden vegetables you eat, this means whole foods – not in cans or pre-cooked and packaged – but the freshest you can get. Start including more of these in your diet. Try eating a vegetable at lunch and at supper. If you already eat cooked vegetables, then try adding a raw vegetable at every meal. Eat real fruits that have not been transformed, cooked, or conserved in some syrup base. Use veggies, fruit, raw seeds and nuts as healthy snack foods to replace the bad snack foods. Carry these around with you at all times.

- **Step 3: Be aware of how food makes you feel physically and emotionally, and keep track of it.** As you experiment with adding more whole raw foods to your diet or with removing junk food, check your dashboard signals:
    - ✓ Are they changing?
    - ✓ Are you getting fewer headaches?
    - ✓ Has your digestion improved?
    - ✓ Do you have more energy?
    - ✓ When you eat more fibre, are you less constipated?

Experiment by taking out certain potentially problematic foods from your diet such as: wheat, dairy, peanuts, eggs, soya, corn or sugar for a two-week period.

- ✓ How do you feel?
- ✓ Are you less lethargic?
- ✓ Do you have more energy?
- ✓ Do you have a better emotional disposition?

Add back in one of these foods at a time and notice what happens over the course of a couple of days.

- ✓ Do you have cramps or bloating?
- ✓ Are you more irritable?
- ✓ Do you feel tired and lethargic?

Once you have identified problematic foods, eliminate them from your diet. As you begin to make these small changes, continue to be aware of what is occurring in your body, and keep noting any improvement.

- **Step 4: Encourage yourself for whatever small step you take to better your health.** Savour these moments. Be proud of yourself. Write this new accomplishment in a journal so that you don't forget. You can refer back to your journal to keep you on track and prevent you from being discouraged and going back to your old ways. No matter how insignificant your action may seem, know that every action is important. This is how you become responsible for your health: one step at a time.

- **Step 5: Be aware of the signs of detoxification.** Your body could go into detox as soon as it starts to get healthy foods. Initially, as you change to healthy food consumption, you might have slight headaches, or your bowels may start to work more than usual. Keep observing. These are most likely signs of detox. These are good signs; be assured they are temporary signs on your way back to health. Make sure you drink a lot of water and add in those exercises to help remove those toxins even more quickly.

- **Step 6: Include a good-quality, bioavailable, well-balanced vitamin and mineral supplement to your diet.** Search for a good, pure supplement that contains no toxic element and is full of antioxidants. Don't forget to include your vitamin D supplement. Also include omega-3 oils to your diet; they have anti-inflammatory properties and help combat the effects of acidity (inflammation) in your body. Notice how the addition of these supplements helps you with resistance, stronger immunity and vitality.

- **Step 7: Start tracking how much water you drink.** Observe if the increased amount of water you drink makes a difference in anything. Are you less dehydrated? Is your skin less dry? Do you need fewer body creams? Are you less constipated? Check your blood pressure regularly and compare the readings. Start analyzing your results. Lack of sufficient amounts of water can make your blood thicker and therefore increase your blood pressure.

- **Step 8: Begin identifying chemical agents and preservatives in your immediate environment.** Verify the labels on all packaged and canned foods. Verify also your cleaning products and your personal care products. Start becoming aware of all the perfumes in your environment as well as other chemicals scents in cleaning products. You will become more and more aware of how these scents are actually very toxic. Notice if your nose feels irritated. Do your eyes water? How do your hands feel after you use harsh detergents? Wear gloves when using cleaners. Better yet, use less of those toxic cleaning products and search for the ones that are environmentally safe. Opt for using good quality personal care products that do not have contaminants like artificial perfumes, parabens or other preservatives in them.

- **Step 9: Check out your emotional state.** Are you angry or really upset? Check if you have buried some negative emotions deep inside. Have you not talked to certain people or family members for a long time because of some un-dealt with issue? Can you put the past behind and forgive and re-establish connection? This doesn't mean that you need to carry on close personal relationships with people who have hurt you, but you must get the tension, bitterness and lack of forgiveness out of the way. Remember, these toxic emotions can wreak havoc in your body with time. Your subtle accumulation of these emotionally generated toxins often becomes greater than your ability to eradicate them.

PAYING THE PRICE

You can prevent degenerative diseases from taking over your body! If you are currently ill or have a degenerative disease, know that it is possible to reverse it and perhaps even heal completely. You now know that processed foods, including all foods that have been chemically altered (junk food), all refined carbohydrates, as well as toxic household and personal care products, all contribute to toxic overload in your body. They will all need to be drastically reduced from your daily intake, as there is a tipping point in which the accumulation of these toxins in your body inevitably begins to be interpreted as disease.

Realize that while we may not be dying from viral diseases so much today, our body burden of toxins is significantly higher than it was 60, 40 or even 20 years ago. This mainly explains why we are now dying from cancer, diabetes and heart problems galore.

Realize that often times it's our addiction that keeps us eating noxious food products, especially refined carbohydrates. It's sometimes hard for us to believe that we can be addicted to products made from wheat flour. However, we really do have a challenge giving them up. If we were asked to not eat any broccoli or lettuce, I don't think we would have that same problem, unless of course we have begun to change to healthy eating habits. After a while, our body starts to crave the good stuff. Take charge of your health and get in the habit of eating a healthy diet that includes a lot of fresh vegetables and a small amount of fresh fruit. Make a conscious effort to begin to listen to and respect your body, and give it what it truly needs to be healthy. Trust yourself. This is within your reach!

NINE MORE ACTION STEPS

- **Step 10: Recognize any temptations and food addictions you may have.** Becoming aware is the first step. Then, try to experiment in diverting those temptations by reminding yourself that you are actually consuming empty calories. There are many ways you can change bad eating habits. Don't keep junk food in your cupboards. It is amazing how creative we can be when we are hungry and only have good, healthy food available to us. Prepare healthy snacks ahead of time, and carry veggies or fruit and nuts with you when you are out and about. You may be pleasantly surprised that the urge to consume a junk snack will have passed. When at an event or party, make a commitment to yourself that before indulging in any unhealthy snack, you will eat a healthy snack first. If you are still regularly eating processed fast foods, make a commitment to always add a salad to your meal. Eat your salad first. Plan your meals ahead of time so that you don't succumb to temptations when you are hungry. Please keep in mind that there may also be an emotional aspect to your food addiction. Get some help with this if necessary.

- **Step 11: Recondition your taste buds and break your addiction to fast foods by doing a short fast or by following a detoxification diet.** It is possible to re-educate your taste buds and actually crave the flavour of whole foods once more. Whole, healthy foods do taste different than processed foods that contain lots of unhealthy fats, sodium and sugar. Crappy food actually impedes your ability to enjoy the true natural flavors of real, non-processed food. At first it takes some adjustment, but if you follow a detox diet – or fast for a few days – you will see that it won't take long before you begin to desire natural, whole, healthy foods. Real food truly tastes good, especially once you have given your body a break from the bad stuff. Experiment with a one-day, three-day or even a weeklong detox. Decide to do this at least two times a year: once in the spring and once in the fall.

- **Step 12: Get in the habit of chewing your food properly.** Consciously slow down. Condition yourself by chewing at least 15 times before swallowing a mouthful; work up to 30 and experiment what it feels like to even do 50. Take the time to relax and chew while eating, in order to allow for proper absorption to take place.

- **Step 13: Work on your morning routine.** Instead of drinking a cup of coffee in the morning, try replacing it with green tea, which contains antioxidants, or simply have a big glass of clean filtered water with the juice of half a lemon added in. Fill a one-quart or one-litre container with clean filtered water and put it on your counter first thing in the morning. Don't go to bed without making sure you have drunk it all. Then work up to two litres. Try starting the day with a nice big green smoothie. The addition of a green leafy vegetable to any type of smoothie makes it a green, highly alkalizing smoothie. Gradually, let go of the commercial juices, soft drinks and caffeinated drinks.

- **Step 14: Respect your natural body cycle.** Don't eat before going to bed. Your digestive system is shutting down and preparing for the restore-and-repair cycle that takes place during the night. If your digestive system is forced to function at night, it can impair this important regeneration cycle. If eating before going to bed is a hard habit for you to break, start your weaning process by eating something light and then replace that by savouring a relaxing herbal tea. Also make sure you respect your body by giving it enough good-quality sleep.

- **Step 15: Become sensitive to your emotional and bodily needs.** Use extra loving care towards yourself when going through a season of difficult times, as when you are mourning for some loss or while going through any other stressful situation. Be less demanding on yourself, and love yourself by taking a break and better care of yourself when you are tired or fighting a cold, for example. Set up good, healthy boundaries. Do not let yourself be the victim of your negligent negative habits.

- **Step 16: Train yourself to not eat when you are angry, hurried or stressed.** These emotions produce stress hormones, which shut down the digestive process. If you eat while in this stressed state, this in turn stresses the body even more.

- **Step 17: Make a commitment to get in some daily exercise.** It can be as simple as parking your car a little farther away from your workplace so that you can walk just a little bit more every day. Or use the stairs instead of the elevator. You can even put a little vigor in your walk. Take every chance you have to move, bend, skip, dance around, twist – keep mobile!

- **Step 18: Honour your body by learning to listen to what it is trying to tell you through your dashboard signs.** This point cannot be repeated enough. Please do not be negligent or put off taking care of your body any longer. You may feel you don't have the time or that it requires too much effort. Perhaps you just plainly have not developed that sensitivity. Or perhaps you would rather avoid facing what's there. Be proactive and courageous, and don't fear the symptoms your body is emitting. Our body wants to heal and can bounce back rapidly if issues are addressed in their beginning stages.

We are living too short and dying too long.

– Dr. Myron Wentz

This truism describes our current, pitiful reality appropriately. However, it is possible for you to die at a ripe old age without having lived the last third of your life crippled, suffering and in pain. By working today to undo our bad habits and gain new ones, we can avoid paying the high price of developing a degenerative disease or living a decrepit old age. Think of these actions as an investment in your old age insurance. It is vital that we start taking steps to undo our often unconscious toxic lifestyle for the benefit of our future physical health.

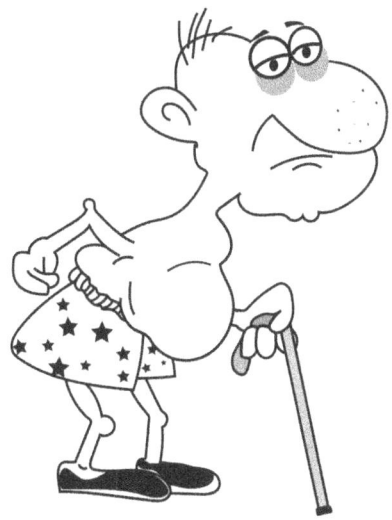

If I knew I was going to live this long, I'd have taken better care of myself.

– Cary Grant

PARTING WORDS

My aim for writing this book has been to help you understand why and how we get sick, and the necessity and urgency of breaking bad habits and addictions to unhealthy foods and reversing our sedentary lifestyles. The ultimate goal being to help you understand the many advantages of developing healthy, new, empowering habits and to motivate you to begin making those changes today so that you can have endless energy and perfect health. This may seem like a daunting task, but now you have the 12 Principles to give you a place to start. Begin gradually and consistently making small, incremental changes, all the while keeping your eyes fixed on the goal of leading a truly healthy energized life. The changes will be imminent.

Getting informed, taking responsibility and changing your habits requires intentionality, especially because doing so goes against the grain of our fast, "everything" society. Develop this winning attitude: "I can't control the rest of the world, but I can master myself. It begins right here and now with me." Making a change in established patterns takes dedication and hard work. Be courageous and vigilant! No longer let yourself be content to remain ignorant to the root causes behind the collective decline of your health. Doctors can't really help us in this area because most of the time they treat only the symptoms. It's an inconvenient truth, but the very food we eat, along with our sedentary lifestyle and products we use in and around our homes and on our bodies, in addition to chronic stress, are making us ill. If we pass on these dietary and lifestyle habits to the next generation we will continue to see the prolongation and worsening of degenerative diseases in our society.

Please do not neglect the primary dis-ease signals your body is emitting just because you don't know what is causing it or because you don't know what to do. You now know better. Many times people fear disease and illness because they fear what might happen to them and so try to ignore it or deny the obvious, often until it's too late. We all are aware of what happens when we neglect to repair small problems in our cars. It just gets worse. Please don't have this attitude with your body, thinking and presuming that your "car" will never break down. Be determined to deal with small, seemingly non-relevant pain or discomforts right from the start. Get help and take action.

Develop the courage to fight for your life, be determined to have great health and to set a good example to those around you. Don't settle for anything less. My hope is that you can live long and healthily enough to be able to pass on to your children and your grandchildren the knowledge and wisdom that you have gained through all of your own particular life experiences: the trials, the tribulations, the good as well as the bad. They desperately need healthy parents, grandparents, and older mentors who serve as good role models and who can guide them in developing sound, beneficial habits in all areas of their lives. Let's do better for ourselves, better for our families, better for our communities and better for our future generations.

I can't guarantee that everyone who eats a healthy diet, avoids as many toxins as possible, exercises regularly, has sufficient amounts of sleep, detoxifies regularly, works on his relationships, works on being positive, doesn't stay stuck in bitterness and anger, develops a spiritual awareness of God and lives a life full of purpose and meaning will not die at an early age. But I can guarantee that those willing to take responsibility to do everything within their reach to live a healthy balanced life will have, what I consider to be, a good life that brings satisfaction with significantly less regret.

As you begin to integrate these changes within yourself, you will also be influencing others to do the same. Start today. Your example will start awakening and inspiring others around you. They in turn may start taking action and eventually they, too, can benefit from having the health and vitality needed to fully live their life's purpose. These people will again inspire others to do the same, thereby also contributing to making this a better world.

May you be blessed in your journey to long lasting great health!

MEET THE AUTHOR

Suzanne Lavoie

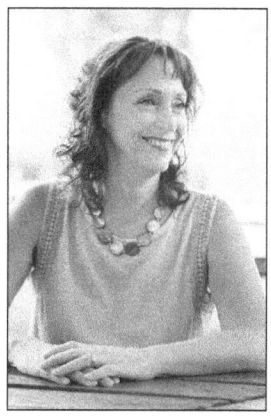

Suzanne Lavoie is a certified Naturopath who graduated from CENAB College, in Montreal, Quebec, Canada, as well as from Trinity School of Natural Health, in Warsaw, Indiana, USA. She has had the opportunity to attend many training sessions and workshops covering numerous topics. Suzanne was trained as a health coach and has also been certified to conduct several emotional healing therapies. She is a natural teacher who also home-schooled three of her four children for both primary and junior grades. She offers conferences and workshops on optimal living, fundamental nutrition, emotional healing and the role of emotions in health.

WWW.SUZANNELAVOIE.COM

WWW.SOYOUTHINKYOUREHEALTHY.COM

Acknowledgements

I want to take a moment to thank some very special people in my life – people who have made this journey possible:

- I am grateful for all of my mentors and teachers I have had over the years, whether through personal one-on-one teachings, group trainings, workshops and conferences or DVDs, CDs and books. Particular thanks to Beth Fodchuk, who many years ago, initiated me to the wonderful world of alternative health. Special thanks to my naturopath teacher Christian Limoges. Thank you for sharing what you know with passion and conviction.

- I am grateful to my dad, who, through his curious nature and child-like sense of wonder, instilled in me the love of learning and discovering new things. Thanks to my mom, who has been a great model of persistence and hard work.

- I am thankful to my husband Michel, who, many years back, took a big risk and stepped out of his traditional job to embark on a new and different career. Because of this, he has given me the financial freedom that has allowed me to follow my passion for learning and to write this book. Thank you also for all your loving support and assistance throughout this whole process.

- Thanks to my kids, for your patience for all those times when I wasn't really available.

- Thanks to my mentor and coach, my brother Roch, for believing in me, affirming me and having the confidence that I had something to offer others. I miss you.

- Thanks to Joshua Rosenthal and Lynsey, and Wendy Walters for providing the support and motivation for writing and publishing this book. Thanks to Kaily Heitz for her support and keen insight, having reformatted my initial writings to make them into an actual book. You did a great job. Thanks to Wendell Anderson, for your professional touch in editing and formatting, as well as your encouragement, and support. Thanks to Erin Hogan for your proficiency and efficiency in re-editing my whole book after having made numerous changes and additions to my original manuscript. A big thanks to Jennifer Coutou Dellar for your support, dedication and assistance throughout the process of fine-tuning my book.

- Special thanks to Wendy from Palm Tree Productions for doing a fabulous job on the cover, interior graphics and layout. Also, to Hasmark Publishing for your professionalism and assistance with my revised version.

- And, finally, thanks to God for always being there with me. He's never been too far ahead of me nor too far behind, but right alongside me, accompanying me every step of the way.

Resources

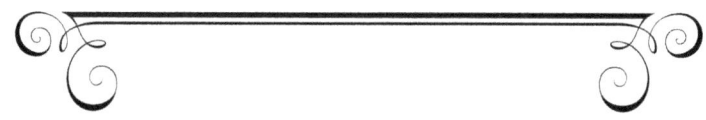

FAMILY FOUNDATIONS INTERNATIONAL
Transforming Hearts, Blessing Generations
8370 W. Coal Mine Ave. Suite 104
Littleton, CO 80123
USA
Phone: 303-797-1139
www.familyfoundations.com

THRIVE
Giving You the Skills to Thrive!
THRIVE Training P.O. Box 2376
East Peoria, IL. 61611
USA
Phone: 309-367-4020
www.thrivetoday.org
www.thrivingrecovery.org
www.joystartshere.com

THEOPHOSTIC
Changing the World One Lie at a Time

P.O. Box 489
Campbellsville, KY
42719
USA
Phone: 270-465-3757
phostic@kyol.net

CARING FOR THE HEART MINISTRIES
Providing Practical Solutions to Specific Spiritual and Emotional Problems

Individuals/Couples Encounter
3545 American Dr.
Colorado Springs, CO 80917
USA
Phone: 719-572-5550
caringfortheheart@msn.com

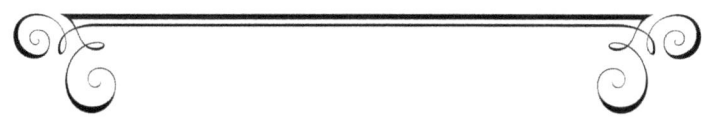

Notes

CHAPTER ONE

1. Mayo Clinic Staff. (2014). "Trans Fat Is Double Trouble for Your Heart Health." Retrieved from http://www.mayoclinic.org/diseasesconditions/high-blood-cholesterol/in-depth/trans-fat/art-20046114

2. Canadian Food Inspection Agency. (2014). "Labelling of Trans Fatty Acids." Retrieved from http://www.inspection.gc.ca/food/labelling/food-labelling-for-industry/nutrition-labelling/additional-information/labelling-of-trans-fatty-acids/eng/1415805355559/1415805356965

3. Center for Food Safety and Applied Nutrition. (2003). "Guidance for Industry: Trans Fatty Acids in Nutrition Labeling, Nutrient Content Claims, Health Claims; Small Entity Compliance Guide." Retrieved from http://www.fda.gov/Food/GuidanceRegulation/GuidanceDocuments-RegulatoryInformation/LabelingNutrition/ucm053479.htm

4. MacWilliam, Lyle. (2008). *Comparative Guide to Nutritional Supplements.* USA: Northern Dimensions Publishing.

5. Davis, Donald R. (2009). "Declining Fruit and Vegetable Nutrient Composition: What is the Evidence?" *HortScience*, 44 (1) 15-19.

6. Scheer, R. & Moss, D. (2011). "Dirt Poor: Have Fruits and Vegetables Become Less Nutritious?" *Scientific American*, 304 (4)

7. Isaacs, Tony. (2008). "Our Disappearing Minerals and Their Vital Health Role (Part 1)." Retrieved from http://www.naturalnews.com/023237_minerals_health_soil.html

8. Ji, Sayer. (2013). "Top Pharma-Brand of Children's Vitamins Contains Aspartame, GMOs & Other Hazardous Chemicals." Retrieved from http://www.greenmedinfo.com/blog/top-us-brand-childrens-vitamins-contains-aspartame-gmos-other-hazardous-chemicals

9 Smith, Jeffrey. (2011). "10 Reasons to Avoid GMOs." Retrieved from http://www.responsibletechnology.org/10-Reasons-to-Avoid-GMOs

10 Campbell, T. Colin, & Thomas M. Campbell II. 2005. *The China Study.* Dallas, TX: BenBella Books. Found in: Hegsted, D.M. (1986). "Calcium and Osteoporosis". 116 (11)

CHAPTER TWO

1 YouTube Movies. (2013, April 24). Food Inc. [Video file]. Retrieved from https://www.youtube.com/watch?v=BtPCtQg51Pg

2 Pesticide Action Network. (n.d.). "Reproductive Health." Retrieved from http://www.panna.org/your-health/reproductive-health

3 Egge, Rose. (2013). "Local Doctors Link Pesticides to Infertility in Women." Retrieved from http://www.komonews.com/news/health/Local-doctors-link-pesticides-to-infertility-in-women-230694311.html

4 Izakson, Orna. (2004). "Pesticides Causing Infertility in the Heartland." Retrieved from https://www.organicconsumers.org/old_articles/food safety/fertility040504.php

5 Schafer, Kristin. (2014). "Pesticides & male infertility: Harm from the womb through adulthood – and into the next generation." Retrieved from http://www.psr.org/environment-and-health/environmental-health-policy-institute/responses/pesticides-and-male-infertility.html

6 Lau, K., McLean, W. G., Williams, D. P., & Howard, C. V. (2016). "Synergistic Interactions Between Commonly Used Food Additives in a Developmental Neurotoxicity Test." Toxicological Science. 9 (1) 178-187

7 Blaylock, Russelll L., MD. (1997). *Excitotoxins: The Taste That Kills.* Santa Fe, NM: Health Press

8 Ibid.

9 NewsMax Media. (2007). *The Blaylock Wellness Report.* West Palm Beach, FL: Christopher Ruddy

10 Blaylock, Russelll L., MD. (1997). *Excitotoxins: The Taste That Kills.* Appendix 1 Hidden Sources of MSG. Santa Fe, NM: Health Press

11 Food and Drug Administration. (2011). "Prescription Drug Products Containing Acetaminophen: Actions to Reduce Liver Injury from Unintentional Overdose." Retrieved from https://www.regulations.gov/document?D=FDA-2011-N-0021-0001

12 Strand, Ray, Dr. (2006). *Death By Prescription.* Nashville, TN: W Publishing Group

13 Houlihan, Jane, Brody, Charlotte, & Schwan, Bryony. (2002). "Not Too Pretty: Phthalates, Beauty Products & the FDA." Environmental Working Group. Retrieved from http://www.safecosmetics.org/wp-content/uploads/2015/02/Not-Too-Pretty.pdf

14 Sarantis, Heather, MS, Naidenko, Olga V., PhD, Gray, Sean, MS, Houlihan, Jane, MSCE, & Malkan, Stacy. (2010). "Not So Sexy: The Health Risks of Secret Chemicals in Fragrance." Retrieved from http://www.ewg.org/sites/default/files/report/SafeCosmetics_FragranceRpt.pdf

15 Ibid.

16 Environmental Working Group. (2007). "Ask EWG: What Is 'Fragrance'?" Retrieved from http://www.ewg.org/enviroblog/2007/12/ask-ewg-what-fragrance

17 McCarthy, Joy. (2014). "Do you know how many toxic chemicals are in your shampoo, your lipstick, your toothpaste?" Retrieved from http://www.theglobeandmail.com/life/health-and-fitness/health-advisor/do-you-know-how-many-toxic-chemicals-are-in-your-shampoo-your-lipstick-your-toothpaste/article21693873/

18 Steckelberg, James M., MD. (2017). "Should I avoid products that contain triclosan?" Retrieved from http://www.mayoclinic.org/healthy-lifestyle/adult-health/expert-answers/triclosan/faq-20057861

19 Health Care Without Harm. (n.d.). "Dangers of Phthalates and DEHP." Retrieved from https://noharm-uscanada.org/issues/us-canada/phthalates-and-dehp

20 Taylor, Paul. (2011). "BPA Being Absorbed from Canned Food: Study." Retrieved from http://www.theglobeandmail.com/life/health-and-fitness/bpa-beingabsorbed-from-canned-food-study/article4252289/

21 Griffith, FD, Stephens, SS, & Tayfun, FO. (1973). "Exposure of Japanese Quail and Parakeets to the Pyrolysis Products of Fry Pans Coated with Teflon® and Common Cooking Oils." *American Industrial Hygiene Association Journal,* 34 (4) 176–178

22 Agency for Toxic Substances and Disease Registry. (2011). "Aluminum." Retrieved from http://www.atsdr.cdc.gov/substances/toxsubstance.asp?toxid=34

23 National Cancer Institute. (2015). "Chemicals in Meat Cooked at High Temperatures and Cancer Risk." Retrieved from http://www.cancer.gov/about-cancer/causes-prevention/risk/diet/cooked-meats-fact-sheet#q1

24 Ibid.

25 Uribarri, Jaime, MD, Woodruff, Sandra, RD, Goodman, Susan, RD, Cai, Weijing, MD, Chen, Xue, MD, Pyzik, Renata, MA, MS, Yong, Angie, MPH, Striker, Gary E., MD, & Vlassara, Helen, MD. (2010). "Advanced Glycation End Products in Foods and a Practical Guide to Their Reduction in the Diet." Retrieved from http://www.ncbi.nlm.nih.gov/pmc/articles/PMC3704564/

26 Luevano-Contreras, Claudia & Chapman-Novakofski, Karen. (2010). "Dietary Advanced Glycation End Products and Aging." Retrieved from http://www.ncbi.nlm.nih.gov/pmc/articles/PMC3257625/?tool=pubmed

27 Canadian Cancer Society. (n.d.). "Chlorinated Water." Retrieved from http://www.cancer.ca/en/prevention-and-screening/be-aware/harmful-substances-and-environmental-risks/chlorinated-water/?region=on

28 Fluoride Action Network. (n.d.). "Water Fluoridation." Retrieved from http://fluoridealert.org/issues/water/

29 Brownstein, David, MD. (2008). *IODINE: Why You Need It, Why You Can't Live Without It*. West Bloomfield, MI: Medical Alternatives Press

30 Fluoride Action Network. (n.d.). "Thyroid." Retrieved from http://fluoridealert.org/issues/health/thyroid/

31 Wentz, Myron, Dr. (2006). *A Mouth Full of Poison: The Truth about Mercury Amalgam Fillings*. USA: Medicis, S.C. 2nd edition

32 Holmes, Amy S., Blaxill, Mark F. & Haley, Boyd E. (2003). "Reduced Levels of Mercury in First Baby Haircuts of Autistic Children." International Journal of Toxicology, 22 (4) 277-285

33 Just, Amanda, MS & Kall, John, DMD. (2017). "Get SMART About Your Mercury Fillings!" Retrieved from http://www.naturalblaze.com/2017/02/mercury-fillings-safe-smart.html

34 Centers for Disease Control and Prevention. (2016). "Immunization Schedules." Retrieved from https://www.cdc.gov/vaccines/schedules/easy-to-read/

35 Holmes, Amy S., Blaxill, Mark F. & Haley, Boyd E. (2003). "Reduced Levels of Mercury in First Baby Haircuts of Autistic Children." International Journal of Toxicology, 22 (4) 277-285

36 Centers for Disease Control and Prevention. (2017). "2017 Recommended Immunizations for Children 7-18 Years Old." Retrieved from https://www.cdc.gov/vaccines/who/teens/downloads/parent-version-schedule-7-18yrs.pdf

37 Centers for Disease Control and Prevention. (n.d.). "Vaccine Effectiveness – How Well Does the Flu Vaccine Work?" Retrieved from https://www.cdc.gov/flu/about/qa/vaccineeffect.htm

38 Canadian Immunization Guide: Part 1 – Key Immunization Information. (2017). "Contents of Immunizing Agents Available for Use in Canada." Retrieved from https://www.canada.ca/en/public-health/services/publications/healthy-living/canadian-immunization-guide-part-1-key-immunization-information/page-15-contents-immunizing-agents-available-use-canada.html

39 Alberta Health Services. (2016). "Influenza Immunization Information if You are Pregnant, Breastfeeding, or have a Newborn." Retrieved from https://myhealth.alberta.ca/Alberta/Pages/Influenza-immunization-for-pregnant-women-and-newborns.aspx

40 Health Canada. (2017). "Mercury in Fish/Consumption Advice: Making Informed Choices about Fish." Retrieved from http://www.hc-sc.gc.ca/fn-an/securit/chem-chim/environ/mercur/cons-adv-etud-eng.php page moved to: https://www.canada.ca/en/health-canada/services/food-nutrition/food-safety/chemical-contaminants/environmental-contaminants/mercury/mercury-fish.html

41 Mercola, Joseph, Dr. & Fisher, Barbara Loe [Mercola]. (2011, October 28). Herd Immunity [Video file]. Retrieved from https://www.youtube.com/watch?v=TFWBelim1Hw&t=297s

42 Safespace Protection and Dimensional Design. (n.d.). "Creating a Healthy Environment in a Toxic World." Retrieved from https://www.safespaceprotection.com/emf-health-risks/what-is-emf/

43 Omura, Y. & Losco, M. (1993). "Electro-magnetic fields in the home environment (color TV, computer monitor, microwave oven, cellular phone, etc) as potential contributing factors for the induction of oncogen

C-fos Ab1, oncogen C-fos Ab2, integrin alpha 5 beta 1 and development of cancer, as well as effects of microwave on amino acid composition of food and living human brain." Acupuncture and Electro-Therapeutics Research, 18 (1) 33-73

44 Puna Wai Ora Mind-Body Cancer Clinic. (2006). "The Theory: By Glen Russell." Retrieved from http://www.alternative-cancer-care.com

45 Ibid.

CHAPTER THREE

1 Jensen, Bernard, Dr. (1999). *Dr. Jensen's Guide to Better Bowel Care.* New York, NY: Avery

2 Walker, Norman, Dr. (1995). *Colon Health. The Key to a Vibrant Life!* Prescott, AZ: Norwalk Press

3 Bragg, Paul & Bragg, Patricia. (n.d.). *Super Power Breathing for Super Energy.* Santa Barbara, CA: Health Science

4 Canadian Liver Foundation. (n.d.). "Liver Facts." Retrieved from http://www.liver.ca/liver-health/liver-facts.aspx

5 Castro, Regin, MD. (2014). "If I have diabetes, is there anything special I need to do to take care of my liver?" Retrieved from www.Mayoclinic.org/diseases-conditions/diabetes/expertanswers/diabetes/faq-20058461

6 Young, Robert & Redford Young, Shelley. (2002). *The pH Miracle: Balance Your Diet, Reclaim Your Health.* New York: Warner Books

7 Ibid.

8 Web MD. (n.d.). "Cysts, Lumps, Bumps, and Your Skin." Retrieved from http://www.webmd.com/skin-problems-and-treatments/guide/cysts-lumps-bumps#1

CHAPTER FOUR

1 MacWilliam, Lyle. (2008). *Comparative Guide to Nutritional Supplements.* USA: Northern Dimensions Publishing. Found in: U.S. Department of Health and Human Services. (1988). Extracts of "The Surgeon General's Report on Nutrition and Health." Washington, DC.

2   Sheeler, Robert D., MD. (n.d.). "Understanding epigenetics." Retrieved from http://healthletter.mayoclinic.com/editorial/editorial.cfm/i/249/t/Understanding%20epigenetics/

3   Mosby's Medical Dictionary, 9th edition. (2009). "Degenerative Disease." Retrieved from http://medical-dictionary.thefreedictionary.com/degenerative+disease

4   World Health Organization. (2017). "The Top 10 Causes of Death: Fact Sheet." Retrieved from http://www.who.int/mediacentre/factsheets/fs310/en/

5   World Health Organization. (2017). "Cancer: Fact Sheet." Retrieved from http://www.who.int/mediacentre/factsheets/fs297/en/

6   Diabetes Report Card. (2012). "Incidence of Diagnosed Diabetes." "Prevalence of Diagnosed Diabetes." Retrieved from https://www.cdc.gov/diabetes/pubs/pdf/diabetesreportcard.pdf

7   Government of Canada. (2015). "Type 2 Diabetes." Retrieved from https://www.canada.ca/en/public-health/services/diseases/type-2-diabetes.html

8   American Heart Association. (2015). "Cardiovascular Disease & Diabetes." Retrieved from http://www.heart.org/HEARTORG/Conditions/More/Diabetes/WhyDiabetesMatters/%20Cardiovascular-Disease-Diabetes_UCM_313865_Article.jsp

9   U.S. Department of Agriculture · Center for Nutrition Policy and Promotion. (1992). "Food Guide Pyramid. A Guide to Daily Food Choices." Retrieved from http://upload.wikimedia.org/wikipedia/commons/0/04/Food_Guide_Pyramid-_A_Guide_to_Daily_Food_Choices_-_NARA_-_5710010.jpg

10 Reymond, William. (2007). *Toxic*. France: Flammarion.

11 Strand, Ray. (2005). *Healthy for Life*. Rapid City, SD: Real Life Press

12 Mercola, Joseph, Dr. (2017). *Fat for Fuel: A Revolutionary Diet to Combat Cancer, Boost Brain Power, and Increase Your Energy*. Carlsbad, CA: Hay House, Inc. 1st edition

13 Puna Wai Ora Mind-Body Cancer Clinic. (n.d.). "The Link Between Cancer and Unexpressed Anger." Retrieved from http://www.alternative-cancer-care.com/cancer-anger-link.html

14 Centers for Disease Control and Prevention. (n.d.). "Physical Activity and Health." Retrieved from http://www.cdc.gov/physicalactivity/basics/pa-health/

15 MacWilliam, Lyle. (2008). *Comparative Guide to Nutritional Supplements.* USA: Northern Dimensions Publishing.

16 Schipper, David. (2015). "Can radiation from mammograms cause cancer?" Retrieved from http://www.consumerreports.org/cro/news/2015/02/can-mammograms-cause-cancer/index.htm

17 Environmental Working Group. (2005). "Body Burden: The Pollution in Newborns." Retrieved from http://www.ewg.org/research/body-burden-pollution-newborns

18 Scientific American. (2010). "Does Mother's Milk Transfer Environmental Toxins to Breast Feeding Babies?" Retrieved from http://www.scientificamerican.com/article/earth-talks-breast-feeding/

CHAPTER FIVE

1 Krolner, Rikke, Rasmussen, Mette, Brug, Johannes, Klepp, Knut-Inge, Wind, Marianne, & Due, Pernille. (2011). "Determinants of fruit and vegetable consumption among children and adolescents: a review of the literature. Part II: qualitative studies." The International Journal of Behavioral Nutrition and Physical Activity. 8 (112). Retrieved from https://www.ncbi.nlm.nih.gov/pmc/articles/PMC3260149/

2 Choi, Candice. (2016). "Just how much sugar do Americans consume? It's complicated." Retrieved from https://www.statnews.com/2016/09/20/sugar-consumption-americans/

3 Lustig, Robert, Dr. [University of California Television (UCTV)]. (2009, July 30th). *Sugar: The Bitter Truth* [Video file]. Retrieved from https://youtu.be/dBnniua6-oM

4 Weight Watchers [Stephanie Vazquez]. (2015, July 8). *If You're Happy* [Video file]. Retrieved from https://youtu.be/mWMsezS1SN4

5 Davis, William. (2011). *Wheat Belly.* Toronto: Harper Collins Publishers Ltd.

CHAPTER SIX

1. Adding protein or fats to processed carbohydrates will help prevent raising your blood sugar to extreme levels but will not necessarily help with the reduction of added toxins or with the addition of healthy vitamins and minerals.

2. Brownstein, David. (2008). *Iodine, Why You Need It*. West Bloomfield, MI: Medical Alternatives Press

3. Mayo Clinic Staff. (2015). "Dietary Fiber: Essential for a Healthy Diet." Retrieved from http://www.mayoclinic.org/healthyliving/nutrition-and-healthy-eating/in-depth/fiber/art-20043983

4. Remer, Thomas, PhD & Manz, Friedrich, MD. (1995). "Potential renal acid load of foods and its influence on urine pH." *Journal of the American Dietetic Association*, 95 (7) 791-797

5. Batmanghelidj, F. (1997). *Your Body's Many Cries for Water*. Vienna, VA: Global Health Solutions, Inc.

6. Moore, Latetia V., PhD & Thompson, Frances E., PhD. (2015). "Adults Meeting Fruit and Vegetable Intake Recommendations – United States, 2013." *Centers for Disease Control and Prevention*, 64 (26) 709-713

7. Drake, Victoria J., Ph.D. (2011). "Multivitamin/mineral Supplements." Retrieved from http://lpi.oregonstate.edu/mic/multivitamin-mineral-supplements

8. Fletcher, Robert H. MD, MSc & Fairfield, Kathleen M., MD, DrPH. (2002). "Vitamins for Chronic Disease Prevention in Adults: Clinical Applications." *JAMA*, 287 (23) 3127-3129

9. Consult the Comparative Guide to Nutritional Supplements by Dr. Lyle MacWilliam for an extensive comparison of more than 1,600 multivitamin supplements.

10. National Sleep Foundation. (n.d.). "Myths - and Facts - about Sleep." Retrieved from https://sleepfoundation.org/how-sleep-works/myths-and-facts-about-sleep

11 Peri, Camille. (2014). "10 Things to Hate about Sleep Loss." Retrieved from http://www.webmd.com/sleep-disorders/features/10-results-sleep-loss#1

12 Cappuccio, Francesco. (2007). "Researchers say lack of sleep doubles risk of death... but so can too much sleep." Retrieved from http://www2.warwick.ac.uk/newsandevents/pressreleases/researchers_say_lack/

13 Darbre, Philippa D. & Harvey, Philip W. (2008). "Paraben esters: review of recent studies of endocrine toxicity, absorption, esterase and human exposure, and discussion of potential human health risks." *Journal of Applied Toxicology*, 28 (5) 565-578

14 National Cancer Institute. (2011). "Formaldehyde and Cancer Risks." Retrieved from https://www.cancer.gov/about-cancer/causes-prevention/risk/substances/formaldehyde/formaldehyde-fact-sheet

SUZANNE OFFERS

Conferences and Workshops

ON VARIOUS TOPICS SUCH AS :

Optimal Living

Fundamental Nutrition

Emotional Healing

And the Role of Emotions in Health

Suzanne also offers Naturopath consultations
and
coaching/counseling sessions online

Please visit

WWW.SOYOUTHINKYOUREHEALTHY.COM
WWW.SUZANNELAVOIE.COM
to receive free downloadable tips and information
that will help contribute to a healthier you.

www.ingramcontent.com/pod-product-compliance
Lightning Source LLC
Chambersburg PA
CBHW060332030426
42336CB00011B/1310